Advance Praise for *Enjoy Every Sandwich*

"A remarkable and unprecedented perspective on life from a doctor living mindfully, adventurously, and even happily with cancer. Lee Lipsenthal lets it all hang out here, and his observations offer us many insights on all the important things in life. Every story, every facet of this healing journey hits home. Rich, heartfelt, and moving. A must-read."

—Martin Rossman, M.D., author of *Guided Imagery for Self-Healing* and *The Worry Solution*

"If you want to learn to love with your whole heart, so that when you come to the end of your life you will have no regrets, Lee Lipsenthal's gracious and caring book is for you. In revealing his own struggles, and doing so with remarkable transparency and responsibility, Lee has not just written a book that is filled with grounded inspiration and hard-earned wisdom. He has written a book that you will never forget."

—John Robbins, author of *Diet for a New America, Healthy at 100,* and *The New Good Life*

"Faced with cancer—and knowing as a physician all too well what his odds are—Lee Lipsenthal does something extraordinary: he digs deep to find wellsprings of humor, gratitude, grit, and inspiration that all of us can use both for our own challenges and for simply living with a newfound joy."

—Rick Hanson, Ph.D., author of *Buddha's Brain: The Practical Neuroscience of Happiness, Love, and Wisdom*

"A heartfelt, inspirational memoir that radiates the hope and courage to overcome adversity. Lee is a physician who understands the necessity of becoming whole and healthy by combining spirituality and science."

—Mitchell Gaynor, M.D., founder and president of Gaynor Integrative Oncology

"Lee Lipsenthal has written a truly beautiful and deeply personal book about living with a life-threatening illness. I highly recommend this physician's account of his Hippocratic life journey into healing himself to all who seek healing and health."

—Michael Lerner, president of Commonweal, cofounder of the Commonweal Cancer Help Program

"*Enjoy Every Sandwich* is a deeply inspiring story of a doctor's response to news about his mortality. Dr. Lipsenthal, using narrative style, shares his engagement with the deepest and most painful of all human emotions—anxiety—and how he has managed his and his family's response to this unexpected and premature challenge. With grace, warmth, humor, and vulnerability, this stricken author encourages and guides the reader to embrace life each moment irrespective of what may be happening. I recommend this book not only to the millions for whom it is personally relevant but for its challenge to all of us to see life as a gift and gratitude as the only appropriate attitude."

—Harville Hendrix, Ph.D., author of *Getting the Love You Want: A Guide for Couples*

"*Enjoy Every Sandwich* by Lee Lipsenthal is a book of heartfulness and wisdom. It is an impressive blend of personal memoir, rich psychological insight, and science. I have been enriched reading it as will anyone else smart enough to do so."

—Frederic Luskin, Ph.D., author of *Forgive for Good*

"This is an amazing, life-affirming, even life-changing book by a man who has learned one of the most difficult of all lessons: how to be himself. In facing the very real threat of his death with utter honesty, deep insight and wisdom, and remarkable humor, Lee Lipsenthal teaches us to appreciate the mystery and glory of our own lives."

—James S. Gordon, M.D., author of *Unstuck: Your Guide to the Seven Stage Journey out of Depression,* founder and director of the Center for Mind-Body Medicine

"At once playful and profound, *Enjoy Every Sandwich* serves up a delicious double-decker. Lee gifts us with gracious guidelines not only for those facing death but for everyone seeking to live life to the fullest. Should be required reading for all!"

—Donald Abrams, M.D., author of *Integrative Oncology,* chief of Hematology/Oncology at San Francisco General Hospital

"This book should be read by every doctor and patient—it is life transforming and affirming. Lee Lipsenthal transitions from doctor to patient to true healer in telling his own journey through cancer and into the deepest acceptance and ease with dying. This is a journey each of us should embrace in our lifetime, and Lee's book is a remarkable guide."

—Stephan Rechtschaffen, M.D., founder of Blue Spirit Costa Rica and Omega Institute, author of *Timeshifting*

"Filled with wisdom, *Enjoy Every Sandwich* reminds us what is really important in life. Dr. Lipsenthal takes us on a journey filled with hope, fear, tough choices, and, most important, love. He reminds us of life's essential ingredients and challenges us to awake to our full potential before it is too late. Thank you, Dr. Lipsenthal, for touching my heart and awakening my soul."

—Mimi Guarneri, M.D., FACC, medical director and founder of Scripps Center for Integrative Medicine, author of *The Heart Speaks*

Enjoy Every Sandwich

Enjoy Every Sandwich

Living Each Day As If It Were Your Last

Lee Lipsenthal, M.D.

Foreword by Dean Ornish, M.D.

CROWN ARCHETYPE
NEW YORK

Published in the United States by Crown Archetype, an imprint of the
Crown Publishing Group, a division of Random House, Inc., New York.
www.crownpublishing.com

CROWN ARCHETYPE with colophon is a trademark of Random House, Inc.

Library of Congress Cataloging-in-Publication Data

Lipsenthal, Lee.
Enjoy every sandwich : living each day as if it were your last /
Lee Lipsenthal.—1st ed.
      p. cm.
1. Cancer—Patients—United States—Biography. 2. Physicians—
United States—Biography. I. Title.

RC265.6.L57A3 2012
362.196'9940092—dc23
[B]
2011026426

ISBN 978-0-307-95515-9
eISBN 978-0-307-95516-6

PRINTED IN THE UNITED STATES OF AMERICA

Book design by Jennifer Daddio/Bookmark Design and Media, Inc.
Jacket design by Jessie Sayward Bright
Jacket photography by Rikki Cooke

1 3 5 7 9 10 8 6 4 2

First Edition

To

my friends and family

who have made this journey worthwhile
and for those who have kept me alive
while on that journey.

And, most of all, to

Kathy

who has been with me through every
difficult step of the past thirty years,
who has held me every night,
and whose love transcends
her need for privacy.
Thanks for letting me tell our story.

Contents

CONTENTS

CONTENTS

Foreword

Imagine the unthinkable: You're a well-known, prominent physician, you have a loving wife and two beautiful kids, and you've made a meaningful difference in the lives of many thousands of people. Your only major unfulfilled desire is to be a rock star, and you're working on that one, too.

In a heartbeat, your life is turned upside down: your doctor just told you that you have metastatic cancer and you probably have less than a year to live.

We all know we're going to die one day; the mortality rate is still 100 percent, one per person. But it's not something we think about very often unless we've had a brush with a life-threatening illness or know someone who has. Even then, though, the awareness of our mortality is hard to hold on to.

For example, people who have recently had a heart attack will do just about anything that their doctor or nurse recommends—change their diet, exercise, quit smoking, etc.—for about six weeks or so, and then they tend to go back to their old habits and patterns of living. Because it's just too terrifying for most people to come to terms with their mortality.

And yet, a fundamental part of many spiritual traditions is a wonderful paradox: to the degree we can embrace our mortality rather than deny it, we can live that much more completely and joyfully. When something profoundly shakes your worldview—like finding out that you have cancer and only a year to live—it radically alters the preconceptions and paradigms of your life.

In this extraordinary book, Dr. Lee Lipsenthal shares his transformative journey with us. Deeply personal yet universal in scope, he eloquently describes how accepting death is intensely clarifying, helping us to understand, to really *know* in every cell, every fiber of our being, what matters and what does not; how we want to spend our precious time, doing what, and with whom. It's not just about how to die peacefully and gracefully; more important, he describes how to live fully.

As he writes, "Being fully alive, I discovered, has nothing to do with the presence or absence of disease." He describes how compassion and forgiveness don't excuse or condone what another person may have done to hurt us, but it frees us from suffering—right here, right now. And when we can apply that same compassion to ourselves—shining a light in the darkness, letting go of anger and judgment—then it frees us and everyone else around us. When a person may have only a year to live, why waste any time holding on to hurts and grievances? And then we realize, "Why should we, either?"

As Quincy Jones said after surviving a ruptured aneurysm that caused bleeding into his brain many years ago, "Live each day like it's your last, and one day you'll be right."

The awareness of death grounds us. It helps us to fend off the advertisements and magazines and well-meaning friends and family who say that having more and doing more is what brings lasting happiness, when we know better.

Preconceptions limit perceptions. Seeing is believing, but we often see only what we believe. Studies show that we are continually filtering our perceptions of how we believe the world is. While this helps to provide a sense of order, it also limits our experiences. Preconceptions can lead to boredom because they limit our experiences so significantly.

Great artists and scientists are able to see the world without filtering it through the veil of their preconceptions and paradigms. They literally see and experience the world in a new way, and then they can share their vision with others, helping to transform the world we experience. This is what Lee does here.

Confronting and accepting death can shatter our preconceptions and shake our beliefs to the core. This can frighten and overwhelm us, or open doors to new, more beautiful ways of living and being that allow us to experience our world anew. Sometimes both. It can even open us to remarkable experiences that don't fit within the conventional scientific worldview, as Lee courageously shares.

I had a near-death experience when I was in college, and it changed my life. I had become profoundly depressed to the point of being actively suicidal. However, once you really come to terms with your own mortality, it's easy to descend into nihilism: why bother, nothing matters, big deal, who cares, etc. That's what happened to me, and it's one of the reasons that we don't think about our own mortality very often.

When I ultimately decided to stay alive, I made a conscious choice to live as fully as possible. Having come about as close as possible to killing myself without actually doing it—staring into the abyss—was liberating.

I decided not to rely on the advice of others on how to live my life, for doing so had almost killed me. So, it became important for me to find out for myself, which meant I was going to lead a messy life. I didn't want to borrow wisdom; I wanted to *know* from my own experiences. I would try a lot of different things, make a lot of mistakes and learn from them. Then, I'd know what was true and what was not. Whatever wisdom I developed would be experienced, not borrowed. As Joseph Campbell once wrote, "I don't have faith, I have experience."

What helped me survive was realizing that an antidote to nihilism is to create meaning in all aspects of our lives. Making every act sacred is what enables us to more fully enjoy life, or as Lee writes, "to enjoy every sandwich."

When I was a teenager, I thought "sacred" meant "boring"—something dry and old, gathering mold and dust. Definitely *not* fun.

Now I understand that "sacred" is just another way of describing what is the *most* special and therefore the *most* fun, the *most* meaningful, the *most* intimate, the *most* erotic, the *most* exciting, the *most* powerful, the *most* sensual, the *most* ecstatic, the *most* playful, and the *most* joyful.

Facing death, we realize that every day is precious, every moment is precious. Realizing this makes everything and everyone sacred in our lives.

Wisdom comes from having the courage to take risks and look stupid, which I have done many times, and to learn from those mistakes as well as the successes. As Lee writes, I began to understand that it's not just how *long* we live but how *well* we live that matters most. And courage comes from realizing that we're here for a very short time, and the biggest mistake may be to play it safe all the time because we think we have all the time in the world. As Fritz Perls, founder of Gestalt Therapy, used to say, "I don't want to be saved, I want to be spent!"

I loved the movie *Groundhog Day,* in which Bill Murray keeps coming back until he gets it right. (It showed on at least a dozen planes I was on when it first came out, which made me begin to feel like I was in the movie . . .) And what Murray gets right is the willingness to take risks, to not stay stuck in a job he hates, to be more compassionate, to learn to play jazz piano—and to take the biggest risk of all: to open his heart fully to the character played by Andie MacDowell.

Because we can be intimate only to the degree we can be vulnerable, but when we're vulnerable, we can get hurt. Your heart is outside your body. Yet everything else is just background music.

A fully committed relationship allows both people to feel complete trust in each other. Trust allows us to feel safe. When we feel safe, we can open our heart to the other person and be completely naked and vulnerable to them—physically, emotionally, and spiritually. When our hearts are fully open and vulnerable, we can experience profound levels of intimacy that are healing, joyful, powerful, creative, and intensely ecstatic. We can surrender to each other out of strength and wisdom, not out of fear, weakness, and submission.

In my life, I've had the opportunity to consult with some of the most powerful and famous people. And if fame, money, and power brought happiness, then they should be the happiest people around. But they're often not; in some ways, it's even more lonely when you come to the end of that myth and find that it doesn't bring you what you thought. At least before they could tell themselves that *if only* they could become so successful, *then* they'd be happy.

That level of success tends to be very lonely; in my experience, once you've achieved a moderate level of success to provide your basic needs, more than that tends to isolate rather than connect. In other words, people are happy *despite* their success, not because of it. What brings happiness is love and intimacy. As Lee writes, "I no longer have a bucket list. I have love in my life."

Ultimately, confronting death inevitably causes us to ask some of the most profound questions: Who am I? Why am I here? Where am I going? What lies beyond? Lee honors the unknown without providing glib answers. He writes, "What is most important to me is that these experiences filled me with questions about life's purpose and mystery," echoing Rainer Maria Rilke, who wrote in *Letters to a Young Poet,* "Have patience with everything unresolved in your heart and try to love the questions themselves."

Death can be the ultimate isolating experience— going into a dark room by yourself forever—or the next chapter in our soul's evolution, like going from one classroom to another, or the river returning to the ocean, becoming one with the source, Thou Art That.

What Lee leaves us with is the profound understanding that we have more choice than we may realize in how we live, and if we live this life well, the next one will take care of itself. This book is Lee's gift to the world, love made manifest.

Dean Ornish, M.D.
Founder and President, Preventive Medicine
    Research Institute
Clinical Professor of Medicine, University of California,
    San Francisco

Enjoy Every Sandwich

Lust for Life

The fear of death follows from the fear of life.
A man who lives fully is prepared to die at any time.
—*Mark Twain*

We all die. This is the nature of life. At some point life ends, but this book is not about that moment. It is about what leads up to that moment. It is about healing the most basic fear all humans share: the fear of dying. It is about the life we can live only after we heal this fear and all the other fears that accompany it: the fear of pain, the fear of loss, the fear of change, the fear of not being enough, the fear of not being loved.

This book is about my journey as a doctor, researcher, and seeker and how I stumbled into a life that transcends this fear that is the root of all our other fears, this fear that causes so much physical illness and emotional dis-ease in our world.

For many years, I was the medical director of the Ornish Program for Reversing Heart Disease. This program is based on a low-fat diet, stress management, exercise, and group support. I had the honor of help-ing hundreds of patients move past their fear of dying into a joy of living. I watched those people become fully alive regardless of difficult health challenges. I watched them enjoy and embrace life even while struggling to walk a few yards with intense chest pain. I watched them dance while I stood by with emergency medical equip-ment. These people had cured their fear of death and led full and dynamic lives. I watched them grow old and saw them play with the grandchildren they thought they would never know. Witnessing all this, I have been deeply inspired by the human drive not just to stay alive but to live fully, love well, and embrace every precious moment of their mortality.

Most people attribute the results of the Ornish Program to a low-fat vegetarian diet. The truth is that these people were not finding a new "lease on life" through broccoli. They were finding a new life by look-ing death in the eye and learning how to turn their way of seeing their lives upside down. They were learning how to connect with others, find inner peace, and laugh again like children. The diet might have helped their heart disease, but the yoga, meditation, and group support saved their lives. I knew this deeply, intuitively, and later statistically through my research. They began to enjoy life so much that the fear of death began to dissipate. It was a remarkable transition. They were no longer dying—they finally were living.

In a practice surrounded by patients enjoying the fullness of life, I began to see many of my medical colleagues as lifeless, struggling to get through each day. They were focusing on the mundane, the hospital politics, the insurance hassles. They were coming home to their families empty, because they had been attempting to care for everyone and anyone they could and ultimately had nothing left for the people they truly loved.

I have spent the last decades of my life helping physicians cure their own fears and step into a life of joy and balance. I have helped them learn to be with each patient in a compassionate way that serves both them and the patient. I also held their hands while they learned to reawaken the parts of their lives that feed their souls. I had the privilege of helping them find the joy of life in their living.

Along this journey, I have had the opportunity to

work with the greatest physicians and healers of our time, learning something new every day. And when faced with my own mortality, I was able to call on and depend on the world's best. But some cures require more than pills, shots, and high-tech equipment. Some cures require a radical intervention of the soul: a change in our mind-set and our way of being. These cures require us to stop racing through our busy lives, working, providing, and consuming. Some cures require that we stop and enjoy every sandwich.

I had suffered from the chronic diseases of our society: fear, stress, depression, and anxiety. This personal experience energized my work researching treatments for heart disease and creating programs to decrease physician burnout. On this path I learned that if my life was full each day, if I enjoyed the people I was with, if I consciously took time to love my family, and if I did work that fed my soul, that day would be a good day to die. Nothing more would be needed. I heard myself repeating this in my workshops and lectures, but I didn't truly know the value and meaning of these words until the day I was diagnosed with a terminal disease. It was on that day that for the first time I knew for sure that the fear of death can be cured. I knew that we no longer have to live with this fear invading our lives in countless ways.

4

I knew that although this fear is based in our need to survive, our other needs—to love, to seek happiness, and to embrace life—are far greater. I knew that life is not just about getting up and going to work. I became one of those patients I had so admired for all of my years in medicine: someone who was dying yet fully alive. After all, we are all dying, some sooner, some later. The real exception is to truly live.

Most important, I knew that I was not born this way. In fact, I was raised in an anxious family that feared death and feared much of life. I realized that I somehow had learned to be at ease with the inevitable: my death. As a lifelong teacher, I knew that anything that could be learned could be taught.

In October 2010, I was honored to be the opening speaker at the American Association of Family Practice annual meeting. I was given free rein to talk about anything I wanted and chose the challenging topic of facing death. It took me four months to write this one-hour talk. I was nervous and excited, but I wanted to get it right. I knew this might be the last talk of my life. I wanted to share the wisdom I had learned: that there is more to life than just managing cholesterol, exercising, and eating well, that our psychospiritual well-being is equally important. Standing in the wings of a massive auditorium, I was about to step onstage in front of four thousand of my colleagues. I was introduced, music swelled, and I was tapped on the shoulder by a "handler." Stepping in front of the lights, I felt like a rock star (my eternal fantasy). I was ready. This was my moment.

For the next hour, I talked about my patients, my colleagues, and my family. I choked on my words because of nervousness and because my salivary glands had recently been radiated. I talked about life, death, and how all of us live in a world of our own imagination that we can barely understand.

As I finished, the audience members rose to their feet in applause. I was stunned, and tears flooded my eyes. I tried to smile, but all I could do was just stand there. Doctors are generally a rather reserved and skeptical audience. They don't give their colleagues standing ovations. It just doesn't happen. I was later told it was the first and only time these doctors ever had. As I left, I was surrounded by my peers—hugged, thanked, and blessed. This, for sure, had never happened at a medical convention. I smiled and cried as one by one I was held in the hearts and hands of strangers and old friends, all of whom now knew the most intimate details of my life and impending death.

I knew then that there was a story to be told. This

book is a culmination of what I've learned. I hope it will open the door for you to embrace your humanity, accept uncertainty, and live a life of gratitude whether you are facing the end now or not. At any moment, in an instant, life as we know it can change. Our mortality waits for us, sometimes patiently, sometimes not so patiently. But it is always there, undeniable and closer than any of us wants to admit. I discovered that my end was nearer than I thought only when I bit into a simple sandwich.

Even death is not to be feared by one who has lived wisely.
—the Buddha

ONE

A Life-Changing Sandwich

On a large enough time line, the survival
rate for everyone drops to zero.
—*Chuck Palahniuk*

On July 19, 2009, I made myself a bacon, lettuce, and to-mato sandwich. As someone who has spent much of his life trying to prevent heart disease, I hate to admit it, but there is something irresistible about the crunch of crisp, cool lettuce mixed with the sweetness of tomato and the saltiness of bacon. I sat down at our kitchen table, a 1950s classic from my grandparents, turned on the news, and began to eat. I had just finished a conference call and was still thinking about that conversation, enjoying the salty-sweet flavors, and watching television all at the same time. After two bites I felt a sudden fullness, as if the sandwich were lodged in my chest. It felt as if I had eaten a golf ball. Pressure and mild pain started to build up in my lower chest. Without thinking, I stood to get some water, and as I swallowed, the water rose up in my esophagus, almost returning to my mouth. Something was wrong. After a very uncomfortable moment, I felt the food and water flush down my throat. As a physician, I knew that the esophagus is very soft and flexible and able to handle a lot, like a balloon that has previously been blown up. Food getting stuck there was in no way normal.

When Kathy came home that night, I told her what had happened.

"It must be a stricture," she stated in her doctor voice. "Forty years of heartburn will do that." She was brushing it off as if it were a nonevent to avoid the more likely and concerning reality.

I have had a hiatal hernia from birth, a condition in which the stomach can slide up into my chest, bathing my esophagus with stomach acid on a regular basis. This can cause significant damage over many years. We wanted to convince ourselves that this was the problem. So I continued in *my* doctor voice: "I'm sure that's all it is. I should get scoped. Who should I call?"

Kathy suggested Tim Sowerby, a gastroenterologist in our community.

Tim agreed to scope me the next day. Being a doctor has its perks.

Kathy and I blissfully entered our world of denial and objective medical talk about what was happening, but below the surface we knew what we were afraid to say out loud. We denied cancer an entrance into our conversation and our lives. I was too young. The problem had just started. There's no cancer in my family. This was just a stricture.

"It's going to be fine," Kathy said. "Tim will dilate it and you'll be as good as new. It's going to be fine."

On the day of the endoscopy, I was a little anxious about the procedure, but I still believed that Tim would find a stricture and dilate it, and that would be all. This was the story that Kathy and I created, and I was sticking to it. I walked the two miles to Tim's office along a beautiful little creek that passes through the small valley towns of Marin County, smiling and nodding to passersby and listening to my iPod. Rock 'n' roll music has always been my constant companion, and this day was no different from any other.

At the gastroenterology suite I joked with the nursing staff as they readied me for the procedure. A quick needle pinch, an IV line, a little fentanyl and versed, and a few minutes later I was out.

On waking, my daughter Cheryl was there at the bedside, reassuring me with her dark, beautiful eyes and loving smile. I had no idea that the procedure was finished. I was still drugged up. I slowly arose out of my haze and waited for Tim to give me a report of his findings. He entered and showed us the photos of my esophagus. In my mind, I saw erosion, but my medical brain was turned off by the medications. Tim said that there was erosion and we should talk in a few days, after he received the biopsy. In retrospect, he was being kind.

Three days passed, and on July 24, 2009, at 5 P.M. I called Tim to see if he had received the biopsy. Deep inside, I knew that I might not have a stricture. I stepped outside and braced myself for the conversation. In his gentle way Tim said, "I do have the biopsy report. Can you come to the office tomorrow so we can discuss it?"

"Tim, I'm a physician; I've used that line before and know what it means. What is it?"

He hesitated, and in that hesitation we both knew what was unspoken. Wanting to talk in the office happens only with bad news. I told him that it was okay to let me know by phone, hoping to make it easier for him, hoping to make it easier for both of us.

"It's an adenocarcinoma of the distal esophagus."

In lay terms, I had cancer of the lower esophagus. At that moment I realized that my life would never be the same. I had a fair idea that this was a really bad cancer. I had never seen a patient live with this diagnosis. I had a 75 percent chance of dying within the next eighteen months and a 90 percent chance of dying within the next five years. It would not be an easy or painless death.

Part of my mind (let's call it my medical mind) kicked into high gear. What do I need to do to complete my workup and treatment plan? What are the statistics today? Which colleagues should I get involved in my treatment? What are the options, if any?

At the same time, part of my mind (let's call it my relational mind) was concerned with breaking the news to Kathy (who would also recognize the gravity of the diagnosis) and our children, Cheryl and Will. Although it was very interesting to witness my medical mind and my relational mind working separately and simultaneously, in that moment I was not agitated or upset. The feeling of calm was unexpected and almost shocking. I sat there peacefully gazing at the trees and wondering why I wasn't upset.

I was fifty-two years old and had just been given a death sentence. It felt strangely acceptable.

Elisabeth Kübler-Ross, M.D., in her now classic 1969 book *On Death and Dying,* described the five stages of emotions that a dying person will encounter. They are denial, anger, bargaining, depression, and acceptance. Every medical, nursing, and psychology student learns these phases. What is not often taught is that they come intermittently, in no particular order, and with a slew of other emotions, many of which occur simultaneously and paradoxically.

A very funny thought-emotion came to me: freedom. I was a chubby teen and have spent my life rigorously watching my weight and exercising regularly. I was never athletic as a child and can remember my shirt buttons straining to stay closed around my waist when I sat. Food was a pleasure that I did not deny myself, and my mother was a great cook. My bad eating habits had led me to develop a career of teaching and researching lifestyle modification to prevent and treat heart disease. We teach what we most need to learn.

At the moment of my diagnosis, all bets were off: no more dieting. I knew that I would be losing weight regardless, so Ben and Jerry, it was going to be nice to renew our relationship! Frankly, I also thought of a direct application of tequila to my cancer, but I knew that I had something critical to deal with first.

I sat in our yard, a peaceful wooded place in the hills filled with the sound of birds, and just breathed in the scent of bay trees and pine. I knew that my life would never be the same—my work life, my family life, and the way I felt physically every day would all be different. I also knew that I couldn't imagine what this would feel like: chemotherapy, radiation, pain, daily nausea, and eventual fading away into death. I had watched many patients experience this but never asked them what it felt like. I was about to find out. I was embarking on a very challenging journey, to say the least. I sat there enjoying the last thirty minutes of my existence before cancer would become the life focus for both my family and me.

The singer and songwriter Warren Zevon died of cancer in 2003. That year, he was a guest on the *Late Show with David Letterman*. Letterman asked him what he had learned in the process of dying, to which Zevon replied, "I learned to enjoy every sandwich." At the time, that struck me as simple and profound. I had used that line in many of my talks about life balance, but it seemed especially relevant to me now, as it was a sandwich after all that had led me to discover my cancer. I laughed to myself.

Then I began to experience helplessness, not for me but for what was about to happen to those I loved. Kathy, my wife and my best friend, would be home soon. Her life was about to change, too, and I could not stop it. She would become a caregiver, watching her husband wither away with illness and eventually die. I wished that I could somehow freeze time so that this conversation would not happen. Our life as we had known it, as we had planned it, was over. After almost thirty years of love, I was about to break her heart in a way that I could never have imagined.

TWO

I Saw Her Standing There (Before I Saw Her Standing There)

The few weeks before the start of medical school I dreamed repeatedly of standing at an altar next to a woman with long, dark hair. I knew that this was my wedding and I knew that the woman was Asian, but at the time I didn't know any Asian women. I had no context for the image of this woman or for the dream that was so real to me that I could reach out and touch it. That was about to change.

On the first day of medical school orientation, I was sitting on a table in the school lobby, a cavernous space filled with the echoes of loudly chatting medical students busily saying hello to one another for the first time. We were all excited and anxious to be there. For most of us this was the beginning of a lifelong dream as well as the end of one competitive journey and the beginning of another. We would be one another's colleagues and competition for the next four years. Some of us would make it; some of us would not. I was talking to one of my new classmates when I noticed a five-foot-tall Asian woman walk in the door. She was wearing jeans, a blue blazer, and Top-Siders. She had long black hair and a bounce in her step. I knew, at that very moment, this was the woman I had dreamed about. It felt strangely obvious, even natural. I was a bit shy about introducing myself to this woman from my dreams, and though I am sure that I did, I have no memory of the first words we spoke to each other. Those words and much of that first meeting were overwhelmed by the excitement of everything that was happening that day. We were not kids anymore—not even college students. We were going to be real doctors.

In the first two years of medical school, we spent six to eight hours a day in one classroom: a large hall with chairs fixed in an amphitheater, our underground windowless center of learning. On day one we settled into our chosen spots, and for two years we barely moved. After all, humans like familiarity. I sat in the second row, on the right, with Mark, Michael, John, and Connie. We would spend most of the next two years together in those seats, taking notes, laughing, and nudging one another if we fell asleep.

Kathy preferred to sit in the back. She was rather shy and did not want to be noticed or called on. Occasionally I would sneak back there just to be closer to her. I laughed as she made funny movements with her lips as she took notes. I found out that she was from Rockville, Maryland, and had gone to Johns Hopkins as an undergraduate and that, much to my disappointment, she had a boyfriend named Richard who lived in Washington, D.C.

I persisted nonetheless (screw you, Richard). We discussed movies and music and various other interests until eventually I asked her to go out with me. This was to be a nondate, two friends going to a movie. I was working this as hard as I could, trying not to seem anxious or overly excited and definitely trying not to appear to want to threaten her existing relationship, although that was my clear intent.

The day before our casual (nondate) night out at the movies, she declined, making a lame excuse about someone visiting from out of town. I knew that she had realized that it was to be a date. She had clearly not seen what I had seen in my dream!

I continued to obsessively persist, with our first date being a quick lunch at a Popeyes chicken restaurant. Not the fanciest of first dates, but I finally got to be with her outside the confines of medical school. Eventually we began studying together, eating together, and occasionally running together.

At the beginning of our second semester, I secretly arranged for Kathy and me to share microscopes in pathology lab. I had worked at the school before becoming a student, so I knew the staff members, who were happy to help me in my romantic endeavors. I knew that lab partners often kept one microscope at school and one at home so they wouldn't have to carry a scope back and forth. If we were lab partners, we were going to be spending a lot of time together in and out of school. I was taking my obsession to new levels.

By the end of the second semester, we were studying together and running together daily and eating many of our evening meals together.

On June 4, 1981, after a run along the C & O Canal in Georgetown, we stopped at the small wooden bridge spanning the canal and rested. It was a very warm spring night, and we were both sweating. Leaning on the bridge railing, inches from each other, we talked. My heart was pounding in my chest not from the run but from what I was about to do. I turned and kissed her. She didn't pull away—she even kissed me back. I will never forget that moment for as long as I live. I had pursued this woman for over a year, and now here I was kissing her on a bridge in Georgetown. Hello, Lee; goodbye, Richard!

My experience of knowing her through my dreams was a prelude to my strange and at times disturbing capacity to see things before they happened. This was to become an increasingly common experience for me over the next few years. Premonitions, or "intuitive hits," as I think of them, are featured heavily in literature and movies. Although these were new and unsettling experiences for me, I came to discover that most people had premonitions but tended to ignore them or brush them off as insignificant.

My love for Kathy felt predetermined. To complete this recipe for destined love, blend in a rush of testosterone (leading to increased libido), a touch of epinephrine (leading to excitement), and a sprinkling of dopamine (leading to contentment), along with the ability to laugh even at the simplest puns, sweetness, competitiveness, physical strength, and a childlike capacity for fun. This was a sandwich I could not possibly pass up.

That October we rented a cabin on the Appalachian Trail and spent Halloween weekend hiking. The fall foliage was breathtaking with brilliant reds, oranges, and yellows, and the air was crisp. On our first night in our rather cheap rental cabin, there were about a hundred flies buzzing around the apex of the A-frame window. We spent the first two hours of our romantic getaway armed with newspapers and a stepladder, committing a fly massacre.

Kathy and I spent every day of that long weekend running and hiking on the trails and each night curled up in front of a wood fire with my German shepherd, JB.

Kathy has a terrible sense of direction, so along our hike, on the second day, near dusk, I lay down at a fork in the trail and told her that she would have to find her way back alone if she didn't agree to marry me. She insisted that I give her time to think about it. To this day, she never decides on anything without thinking about it for a few days and then only when pressured.

That night, in the cabin, after an evening spent drinking wine and carving her first Halloween pumpkin, Kathy agreed to marry me with the odd caveat "as long as we don't tell anybody." She is an intensely private person and didn't even want our classmates to know that we were dating (although they all knew). This was a side of her that I didn't understand at all. I am gregarious and revealing at the drop of a hat. She wanted to keep our private life private. She also felt that it was irresponsible for two students still on the "parental assistance plan," PAP in my language, to be planning to marry. I have never let responsibility get in the way of love and pleasure, and my brain was soaked in hormones. How could logical thinking counter the swirling mess of chemicals that was my brain in love?

Later that year, I borrowed money from my father to buy Kathy an engagement ring. It was a student-size diamond on a modest gold band, and to this day I haven't paid him back (but he says it's okay). For days, I would take it out of its blue box and hold it in my hands. I was overwhelmed with anticipation and impatience. On January 14, 1983, I made reservations at L'Auberge Chez François, a quaint and very expensive (for medical students) restaurant in Great Falls, Virginia. It was so popular that you had to call a month in advance to the day to get a table. I felt lucky to have gotten one.

On February 14, there was a significant snowstorm. I was anxious about missing our reservation but even more nervous about my "official" proposal. Kathy had no idea where we were going or what I was up to. Finally, after traveling an hour in the blinding white storm, we arrived for our very special, very unaffordable dinner. The restaurant looked like an old house, and they had a roaring fireplace. It was all very romantic. After we finished our main course, I presented her with the ring and again asked her to be my wife. She smiled and cried and said yes. I asked her if I could tell the world, and she agreed. I can still sit here today and remember the joy and the look on her face and feel the love in my heart. I have relived that moment in a restaurant in Virginia on a cold winter's night thousands of times in my mind over the last thirty years.

That August we were married.

This July I had to tell her I was dying.

THREE

Two Doctors Enter the Valley of the Shadow of Death

Sitting by the pool, my head was spinning as I pondered the conversation I had to have with Kathy. Although I've had this conversation with patients numerous times, I never fully understood the heart-wrenching intensity of having to tell one's family the bad news. This conversation would shift the direction of our lives forever. On this warm summer evening our old life would end and a new one, focused on dying, would begin.

I heard her car pull in and went to the bedroom. It was my safe haven and the place where I knew I wanted to be when I told her. She came in the front door, and I stepped out to meet her.

"Hi, can you come in? I want to talk." I motioned to the bedroom.

She knew something was wrong. "Come into the bedroom" was reserved for serious conversations.

"We need to talk; come sit." I motioned her toward the bed.

"What's wrong?"

"I spoke to Tim today. He got the path report back."

She stared at me, fear in her eyes.

"It's cancer."

Kathy started to cry and held me tighter than she had ever done before.

For long minutes, we sat there, saying nothing and holding each other as life as we knew it, as we planned it, shattered around us.

"I want you to know that whether I live or die from this, I'm okay with it."

I'm not sure why I said that. I did want her to know that I was all right, but it must have seemed insensitive to her. She was not ready to hear that her husband was okay with dying! Knowing the Kübler-Ross stages of dying, she said, "You can't go right to acceptance!" She was angry that I was at peace. And in her mind, I was giving up, accepting death, and planning to leave her.

Kathy went into battle mode. "You're going to be fine. You'll get through this. You're young and in good shape. It's going to be okay."

I couldn't fall into such certainty and understood it was just a defense mechanism. All I could say was, "We'll see." I didn't know if I would be fine or not. I just knew that I had a lot to do.

In a flash, we both switched into doctor mode. We began to think and plan, decide whom we needed to consult with, and we decided to go online and find out what treatments were available. In retrospect, it amazes me how quickly we doctors can do this—shut down intense human emotion, even when it is about our own lives, and drop into a state of doing and planning. It is far easier than dealing with the emotional pain, and we do it well.

"What will you do?" she asked, knowing that I needed to see if the cancer had spread.

"I'll schedule an appointment with Marin Oncology, start the workup process, and get opinions from our friends and colleagues."

"I guess we'll cancel England." We had a trip scheduled in two weeks to go to the UK with our kids. She wanted me to move to treatment right away.

"No, I want to go. If this is our last family trip, I want to enjoy it off chemo."

Again, this did not sit well with her. She wanted me to dive right into the workup and treatment without delay. "We'll talk about it," she said. The discussion was not over yet.

Kathy was getting upset that I was so nonchalant about the whole thing. She wanted me to say, "I'm going to get this worked up, switch to a raw food diet, bike a thousand miles, and beat this thing. Screw vacations; I'm going to live!" But I didn't feel that way. I just wanted to enjoy whatever life I had left. I didn't have "fight," and this pissed her off, so we dropped back into practical matters.

"What about the kids? When should we tell them?" I was supposed to take Will, our eighteen-year-old, to his college orientation in Southern California in two days.

Kathy thought we shouldn't tell our kids until we returned. She didn't want to ruin his excitement over college.

I agreed. "Then we can't tell anyone. I don't want the kids finding out until we tell them."

She agreed. I would quietly make my medical appointments but tell no one until the next week.

We spent the night online sitting across from each other, both of us on our laptops, studying the world medical literature on esophageal cancer. We searched every review article we could find: 90 percent death rate. We looked at national databases on treatment recommendations and outcomes: 90 percent death rate. We dove into studies from India, Japan, and Germany: 90 percent death rate. We searched the National Institutes of Health's database for ongoing studies. There were none. We were getting depressed and exhausted. Hopelessness set in.

Kathy usually goes to bed after me, but this night I asked her to come to bed early and hold me. We had some wine and held each other, talking about issues that we could control—what I would do with work, disability policies, how we would pay for Will's college, and other business around how our lives would change. It was far easier to focus on those issues than to talk about my 90 percent likelihood of dying.

We hold each other off and on through most nights, but on this particular night there was a sense of desperation. Kathy held me all night long as if that would keep the inevitable at bay. She held on to me so that I wouldn't leave her.

Over the next day we looked at all the various

treatment options, both mainstream and alternative. I felt very calm about it. We were in doctor mode and emotionally shut down.

"I'll e-mail Mitch Gaynor, Andy Weil, Dean, Donald Abrams, and others and gather their opinions." I had a great network of friends I could turn to for information and advice.

"How about going to see Amma [the Indian spiritual leader] or John of God [a Brazilian healer]?" she pleaded, looking for miracles when there were none to be found in the medical literature. There was desperation in her voice.

"No, I'll do surgery if I can, chemo, radiation, and meditate. I'll call Marty about acupuncture, and I'll use whatever herbs Andy, Donald, and Mitch recommend."

Kathy could not accept that decision. Here I was, with access to a world of spiritual healers, and I was going to sit at home, take supplements, and meditate. My wife needed me to fight cancer, yet I could not find fight in me. She wanted me to do anything and everything to avoid dying, but my intuition told me to just get quiet, shut down my busy life, and meditate. It's not that I had given up; it's just that I had no agitation or anxiety, which provides the energy needed to fight and to endure extreme treatments. I had no fear. Let me be clear: I was not going to sit back and do nothing about the cancer. I loved my life and clearly preferred to live, but I did not fear death.

For years I'd been teaching that "today should be a good day to die." This is a Native American expression sometimes used in battle. Today I die for a good cause, but it also can mean that if each of our days is lived fully, without remorse, with love and service, any day is a good day to die. My life up to that moment had been full of love, laughter, great music, learning, and teaching; a wife I loved and admired; and kids I was proud to be with. I had a profound sense of connection with spirituality, something out there bigger than myself. I had enjoyed many great sandwiches already. If I died today, I would have had more than enough to satisfy me.

It may strike you as odd that I could have so much gratitude for this life that I was about to lose, but I had approached my life a bit differently than most. Every day for the last twenty years, I have practiced gratitude. I started by thinking about the things I was grateful for on a daily basis, writing down things that I was grateful for on a nightly basis, reminding myself of how lucky I was. Later, I began to use gratitude in my meditation practice.

Gratitude became a small practice with a big payoff. In fact it is a vital part of savoring this sandwich of life.

I was not born with this mind-set, growing up in a family that treated every death and illness as if it were a tragedy, and was trained by a medical community where death was the enemy. Yet for me, July 24, 2009, was, simply, a good day to die.

FOUR

From Neurotic to Knowing

Not a shred of evidence exists in favor
of the idea that life is serious.
—Brendan Gill

How does an anxious guy from New Jersey become a guy who can learn to accept even death?

I was raised in an upper-middle-class northern New Jersey town filled with brown and beige two-story homes, two middle schools, and a high school. My father was a dentist, and my mother a schoolteacher turned stay-at-home mom. It was a typical postwar family for a late baby boomer to grow up in. Success in that community was to go to college and then move on to a professional school. In that world, being a doctor or lawyer was expected.

However, there was quite a lot of anxiety in my household. My parents seemed to worry a lot about everything. Not quite the Woody Allen level of anxiety but not too far from it. Everywhere I went, I was taught to lock doors behind me, look over my shoulder while walking in the street at night, and leave nothing visible in my car. We worried about whether it would snow or rain. We worried about everyone's health, even relatives I didn't know at all. My father would tell me (and does to this day), "There are people out there who want to hurt you." I still don't know who these people are. I know they must be there; Daddy told me so.

My parents see the world as a dangerous place. They convince themselves that they are at risk most of the time. This is reinforced by the stories they tell themselves and each other. My friends Nita Gage and Shannon Simonelli and I have come up with a word to describe this world that we create in our minds—our Neuroimaginal™ world. This is the world all of us convince ourselves is true.

I understand that my parents are of a very different generation. I understand that they grew up in New York City, where crime is more common. I understand that they grew up in a world where people actually killed you because you were Jewish. Maybe they came by their anxieties honestly, but they honed them to an art.

My sister and brother have both struggled with anxiety and depression issues throughout much of their lives. My role was to be the one who made light of it all with humor, but I carried an underlying anxiety into my adult life. What if I didn't get into professional school? What if I wasn't a success? In college, I often curled up in my small part of the dorm room and put on headphones to try to relax. There was something inside me that made me uncomfortable in my own skin.

Going to rock concerts helped me get out of this anxious state and into a state of pleasant postconcert fatigue. The buzz of a great band and the feeling of the bass drum and guitar's sound waves vibrating through my entire body were transformative to my early stressed-out brain. Venting, vibrating, and dancing were my way of dealing with anxiety. Jumping up and down with headphones on and playing air guitar had a major soothing effect on my nerves. It was how I self-medicated. I did draw the line, however, at singing into air microphones—a guy has to maintain his standards.

I was far more interested in music and hanging out with my friends than I was in school. This led to a B average, which at the time was enough to get me into a good college in Washington, DC.

Premed and prelaw students surrounded me. In that

atmosphere, going into medicine seemed like the right and admirable thing to do. My grade-point average, however, was not stellar. Somehow, hanging out in the DC rock 'n' roll scene did not improve my GPA. My first year of applying to medical school consisted of over fifty applications and just as many rejection letters. I guess they weren't looking for anxiety-prone air guitarists.

In response, I began to "tune myself up." I exercised an hour and a half to two hours each day (to the point of obsession). I put myself on a rigid diet to maximize my health. I enrolled in a one-year master's program in human physiology and earned a 4.0 average. I became a lean, mean study machine. I used all of my Type A behaviors to their fullest. What did this get me? Fifty more med school rejection letters!

I knew I needed to find work that would enhance my chances of getting into medical school and provide a backup career if I didn't get in (I was obsessed but not stupid). I decided to work in a science lab and was lucky to land a job working with a neuroanatomy teacher, Sal Rapisardi, at Howard University in DC.

This was a great year of learning science, studying, and learning how to write scientific papers. I continued my fitness quest with running and weight lifting. I became part of the affiliate teaching staff and got to know the faculty quite well (which, as you have seen, served me well in my quest for Kathy's attention). I still kept the applications flowing and continued to get rejection letters. My desire to become a physician increased proportionately to the number of rejection letters I received, so I began to apply to medical schools in other countries.

Two weeks before leaving for a medical school in France, I received a call from the dean's office of Howard University telling me that I had cleared the waiting list and had been accepted into Howard's medical school. I still don't know who, if anyone, pulled the strings (probably Sal), but after three years and over a hundred applications, I was in.

In medical school I excelled academically. In my three years of applications to school, I learned self-discipline—how to eat, exercise, and study—all of which served me well in the rigors of medical education and later in my career teaching patients about healthy lifestyles. I sat in the front of the class, wanting to catch every word and not fall behind. Anxiety led to a high need for control, which turned me into a discipline monster. I studied late every night, ran every day, and used music as my release. Headphones on, world gone.

I did notice something unusual: If I crammed information into my brain for about twenty minutes and then cranked up one great three- to four-minute rock tune and danced around, the information would stick, so I got into the habit of twenty minutes of studying and four minutes of rock 'n' roll. I know now that what I was doing was managing my stress hormones. When I rocked out, my stress hormones would drop. This combined state of lower stress and greater energy increased my thinking brain's, or cortex's, function, thus improving my memory and learning. Rock 'n' roll and a good run each night helped me succeed in medical school. I believe I graduated third in my class thanks to the Ramones and an old pair of Nikes.

Night call at the hospital as a medical student was a crazy time. Late at night the world of the hospital became a strange and scary home: dead bodies in the morgue, pain and suffering in the ER, and visiting with grief-stricken and worried families trying desperately to believe that it was all going to be all right.

There were two places of refuge: the cafeteria for coffee, ice cream, and other treats and the call room for sleep and rest if you were lucky enough to have twenty minutes to lie down. At 3 A.M. one night, I went to the call room for a short rest, and as I stumbled in and flicked on the light, my classmate Tony was sitting there, meditating. How could he sit there at 3 A.M. in the middle of a busy hospital, in the dark, and somehow be at peace? I would be lying there awake thinking of the next admission, what lab tests did I forget, which attending would yell at me in the morning, or which patient would crash next, yet Tony was chillin'. I wanted what he had.

The idea of meditating was not a foreign concept to my generation. The Beatles had gone to Rishikesh, India, to study with the Maharishi fifteen years earlier. As a rock fanatic, if it was cool for the Beatles, it was cool for me. I even tried to meditate a few times when I was a teen but never had any training. At the age of twelve, I began sitting and breathing, sometimes in silence, sometimes listening to music (Mike Oldfield's *Tubular Bells* and the music of Tangerine Dream were favorites). Music and my amateur form of meditation helped me deal with my underlying anxiety and tendency toward depression. I continued some mild forms of meditation off and on through high school and college, but not as a daily practice. I just didn't know how to do it, but now, in the middle of medical school craziness, it was a very attractive idea!

Did I follow through? Not really. I could have signed up for a meditation class or purchased some tapes or books to learn from, but I didn't. I just continued to be anxious, to dance, and to run. My system was working for me, my grades were great, and I didn't want to screw it up.

If medical school was stressful, residency was *Death Race 2000*: sleepless nights, crazy patients in the emergency room, death and trauma, people losing loved ones, and utter exhaustion. Add to this a new marriage and a first child (born during medical school), and I was toast.

Something happened to me in my last year of residency that gradually and subtly changed my life. Phil Weiser, a Ph.D. exercise physiologist, was running the hospital's pulmonary rehabilitation program. I was very interested in cardiac rehab, so in addition to his pulmonary rehab program, we began a small cardiac rehab program at the hospital. It was there that Phil taught me the benefits of stress management for heart and lung patients. Now meditation was not just what the Beatles and Tony did; meditating enhanced health and improved longevity. I began to learn meditation in earnest in order to teach it to patients.

I started with simple recorded, guided meditations based on mindfulness and loving-kindness practices. I would choose one in accordance with my mood that day. If I was anxious, mindfulness seemed to help. If I was upset about something in a relationship, loving kindness was the ticket. Each day I would sit and listen for twenty to thirty minutes as I followed the guided meditation. For me, starting in the morning worked best (I am a morning guy), but I also supplemented this with evening meditation. I gradually, over many months, built a practice that was sustainable.

The challenge to change, for me personally, began after my residency. I was a practicing physician, happily married and the father of two children. The wake-up call occurred while riding the trolley to my office in Philadelphia, and I was struck with a full-blown panic attack. I became agitated, restless, and sweaty. I thought I was going to pass out. I thought I was dying, and I didn't know why. I was three years out of residency, working in a downtown, corporate, suit-and-tie medical practice. As an internist with a strong interest in lipids (cholesterol) and cardiovascular prevention, I spent most of my days seeing individuals who were interested in decreasing their risk of heart attack and stroke. A noble calling, but on that particular morning, bumping along on a rickety trolley car track, the thought of hearing myself say "low-fat diet, exercise, manage stress, take your medications" twenty to thirty times over the next few hours became unbearable. I thought I was going to be the one with the heart attack. The routine of medicine and the repetition of my own words were driving me crazy.

Those outside the medical field believe that the stress in medicine comes from dramatic events such as the ones they see on TV. For most physicians, that level of excitement and challenge is fun and satisfying. More stressful for clinicians are the routine, mundane, day-to-day occurrences such as paperwork, phone calls, dictating or typing charts, and repeating the same information over and over to people who may be only half listening or half understanding. The other major stressor for physicians is our own personality structure. We are a pretty screwed-up group—obsessive, perfectionist, and Type A to the core. The routine of medicine was killing me. The lean, mean discipline machine I'd created in medical school was leaking at the gaskets.

Kathy and I had two children, two jobs, outside responsibilities (I was the chairman of a local school board), and too much in our lives. By all external standards, I was a success, yet I was in a constant state of panic and depression.

Over the next few months, I started myself on Prozac. I was depressed and stressed and couldn't see outside this world I had created for myself. I felt imprisoned in this tiny box of life, which was supposed to be so wonderful. I was living the life I had envisioned as perfect. How could I, the smart, funny, exercising, *meditating* doctor with the sweet wife and family, be so miserable?

I didn't think medicine was supposed to be boring or routine. "It wasn't supposed to be like this!" I told myself. I was burning up my energy whining about what the practice of medicine was *supposed* to be like and not enjoying what it really *was* like. What I was yet to learn was that my *perceptions* were at the root of my anxieties.

I held a false image of what adult life should look like. I thought that we would be financially well off, that we'd have great vacations and a nice house, and that I would come home to a happy, loving family. I didn't know that we would be struggling financially and driving an old car and that I would come home to a fatigued wife and the shared demands of family life. The reality of my world didn't match my Neuroimaginal construct of what life was supposed to be like. My misperceptions of how life was supposed to be had left me tired, angry, anxious, and depressed. This was the first key to recognizing what needed to change, but I still needed a larger kick in the pants to motivate me toward real change.

FIVE

When Your World Collapses

In my early thirties, my beliefs about how my life was supposed to look were killing me. I continued to meditate and to study Eastern philosophy, emotional intelligence, and neurophysiology. At first I acquired this knowledge in order to teach it to my patients, but through this process, I began to realize that I was the one who needed help. I realized that it wasn't the world doing me wrong—I was harming myself. If, in my dad's language, there was someone out there trying to hurt me, it turned out to be me and my view of life.

I began to take yoga classes with my patients and to study the science of yoga and meditation. These new techniques, practices, and studies began to give me a sense of release from the confining box in which I was living. I didn't know where it would lead, but it felt good to be pushing and scratching at the box's walls.

My anxiety slowly began to fade. I noticed that the less anxious I was, the more clearheaded and creative I became. I learned that this was a physiological effect. Brains bathed in stress hormones do not function as well as stress-free brains. I also discovered that along with my meditation, exercise would help me sleep better and think more clearly. Most important, I began to learn that the goal was not in the doing but in the being. As the Buddhists say, "Before enlightenment, chop wood, carry water. After enlightenment, chop wood, carry water." I needed to learn how to live within my daily routine with clarity and happiness and understand that the end result would be authenticity and a sense of connection with purpose and meaning. I realized that the challenge was not learning how to be a great doctor but learning how to live a great life while using my medical skills and knowledge. I needed to pay attention to my soul's calling.

On this journey, I read Dean Ornish's book about reversing heart disease by using yoga, social support, exercise, and a vegetarian diet. As I read the book, I recognized Dean's voice as my own. It was eerie to read what sounded like words coming from my own mouth. Somehow he brilliantly put into words and demonstrated

44

through careful research what I had been thinking and saying to my patients. I knew that I would work with him someday.

This felt like a soul's calling that could not be ignored. I could find purpose within my career of medicine. I didn't have to give up being a doctor to be happy. I contacted Dean, telling him I would be in San Francisco and would like to meet with him. In reality, I had no other reason to be there. I lied, but I knew I needed to meet him. We talked for some time, and I shared that I had been treating patients in Philadelphia, using yoga, meditation, group support, and low-fat diets. He was thrilled that I was having this much success with a similar approach to heart disease. He was just beginning to offer retreats for heart patients and asked if I would like to staff them and run the medical aspects of the program.

Over the next few years and many of those weeklong retreats, I became more invested and involved in this holistic way of treating patients. I also learned how to teach and loved it. Getting up in front of an audience became easy and fun. Four times a year I would fly to California to be the medical director of the Ornish retreat programs. Then I would fly back to Philly to "chop wood and carry water," continuing the routine of my everyday life.

Then Destiny/God/Spirit or just plain luck stepped in. At that moment, however, it didn't feel like luck.

We owned a three-story town house that had been built in 1895. It had beautiful oak floors, bay windows, and carved wooden fireplaces. Our neighbor who owned the adjoining house was digging out his basement. He did not shore up the foundation properly first.

On a quiet Saturday morning while Kathy was seeing patients at the hospital and I was home with two-year-old Will and eight-year-old Cheryl eating Cheerios, there was a thunderous roar. I felt and heard a wall come down like in an earthquake. Workmen came banging on our front door and told us to get out immediately. Our neighbor's three-story house, which adjoined ours, had crumbled to the ground, and our house was rendered unlivable. I sat on the curb with the kids still in their pajamas. The police and fire departments rushed in to cordon off our home. We were homeless, with no access to our possessions.

The next day Dean and I were speaking, and I told him what had happened. He said, "Does the message need to be any clearer? Move to California." After much shuffling and months of legal battles with insurers, we were off to California. It was the universe pushing me to overcome my fear of change. I was now the medical director of the Preventive Medicine Research Institute.

What this move also led to, and maybe most important, was deep personal relationships with many great therapists and yoga teachers who worked with the institute. This helped deepen my practice and personal growth immensely. Through desiring the health benefits of yoga and meditation, I also began to experience the spiritual benefits. I gained a greater sense of connection with things outside myself. I also developed a keen intuition, knowing without knowing why. I was in touch with my inner wisdom, what you might call my knowing self.

I also learned something profound. I couldn't "manage" stress. Stress was just my response to life's events. Stress wasn't something to be managed. Once it happens, it has happened. My parents taught me to look for stress in life. I now realized that looking for stress creates stress. The harder I looked, the more I found. What I could begin to do now was shift my perspective on life events.

I also began to learn how little control I had over life events and how sometimes a curse becomes a blessing. I learned gratitude in light of adverse events or circumstances. My house crumbled to the ground, and I came to see it as lucky. Most people I speak with have experienced significant hardships only to view them later as positive events or maybe even a gift from God.

If I looked for fun, joy, and playfulness, I would find fun, joy, and playfulness. If I looked for trouble, stress, and heartache, that was what I would find. I found that if each night I wrote down or told Kathy three things that I was grateful for, each day was filled with more fun and joy. Fear and anxiety began to fade. I also found acceptance of the stressors of life as a part of life, and in that acceptance I found peace. My Neuroimaginal worldview had grown larger. This would serve me well twenty-five years later when I was dealing with cancer.

SIX

Sitting Down and Shutting Up

Put your ear down close to your soul and listen hard.
—Anne Sexton

My newly adapted practices of meditation and yoga began to change my life and attitude. I was less grumpy, I yelled at our kids less frequently, I enjoyed my work more, and I no longer felt the agonizing pressure of discord in my soul.

I also, through my reading and practice, became very aware of the health benefits of meditation. I knew that the greater our sense of peace is, the better our hearts, brains, and immune systems function. Just check your pulse while taking a few deep breaths and feel it slow down.

It was these discoveries that led me to increase my

meditation practice when I was diagnosed with cancer. I knew that the more I meditated, the healthier my bodily systems would be and the better I would be at resisting the growth of cancer cells. I also knew that it would help me deal with the emotional issues that would arise in treatment as well as manage the pain and nausea that happen with chemo and radiation. Meditation has always been my most powerful drug.

If there was a drug that changed lives in this way, without side effects, I bet you, hands down, it would be the biggest-selling drug on the planet, yet it is available to all without a prescription, and, oh yes, it's free. So why doesn't everyone meditate? Because meditation works only if practiced on a nearly daily basis and practice takes time and commitment. How do you get to Carnegie Hall? Practice, practice, practice.

Some people feel that meditation has some religious connotation. Many religions use meditation, but some just call it prayer. Some say prayer is talking to God or the universe and meditation is listening to the answer. There is really no difference. If you prefer to pray, do so every day for twenty to thirty minutes. I do suggest that you pray not for what you want but to thank God for what you have, a prayer of affirmation.

Have you ever sat quietly on a beach, hypnotized by

the waves, the vastness of it all? Have you ever played music or gardened or practiced a hobby and suddenly realized that just for a moment you had forgotten where and who you were? Have you ever prayed and felt a sense of connection with something bigger than yourself? These are meditative moments, moments when your thoughts are quiet enough that you are just you—alone and in peace—and that is enough.

When I teach my fellow physicians about meditation, I encourage them to enjoy these moments and pay attention to how they feel while sitting in this place of peace or awe and to spend an extra few minutes in this state before moving on to their next activity, event, or thought. Just sitting, breathing gently, and paying attention to how they feel, what they hear, and what they see. Trying not to judge any of it as good or bad, right or wrong, just accepting it for what it is. This is mindfulness.

In the language of psychology, these are transpersonal moments. In the language of religion, we are connecting with God or Spirit. In the language of neurophysiology, we are changing the balance between epinephrine, norepinephrine, dopamine, and serotonin (the stress and relaxation hormones). Over time, we are also changing the brain's anatomy, which enhances our focus, concentration, and awareness.

Meditation diminishes fear and anxiety by affecting the function of our fearful survival brain. This part of the brain is a potent source of fear and self-protective behaviors. It exists to help us rapidly assess and respond to potential danger. For many of us, it becomes hypervigilant (always watching) and out of balance with the rest of the brain. An extreme example of this is obsessive-compulsive disorder, in which almost everything is perceived as a threat. This hypervigilant state forces the individual into overevaluation (obsession) and creates a need for the person to try continually to create safety through routine or repetitive behaviors or actions (compulsion). The person may be consciously aware of these abnormal behaviors but can't regulate or control them.

The survival brain is also the root of our fears of death, the ultimate threat to survival. When the survival brain is too pumped up, the fear of death pervades our lives by decreasing our desire to take risks and try new things. We become limited in what we can create or experience because of our fear of taking risks. Life becomes a fear-based trap.

Our connection with and support of one another help communities survive adversity. We see this clearly during tragedies such as September 11, 2001, when the entire nation became a community intent on surviving. We were all at risk for that brief moment, and we became one. A fear-based life that is not shared with others decreases our ability to connect. When people are alone in their fears, they tend to isolate themselves, cutting off the human instinct to gain support. This leads to loneliness, depression, and despair.

Fear can be a nasty little prison to live in. Meditation can be the key that unlocks the prison door.

The change, through meditation, occurs in the anterior cingulate cortex, which serves as a check-and-balance region for the survival/emotional brain. I like to think of this as our inner guru, the part of our brain that serves as the wise overseer of life events. When something is perceived as dangerous, the survival/emotional brain checks in with the guru brain, which either supports or diminishes the stress response. The guru brain tells us whether the stress reaction is appropriate, given the situation. With meditation, the pathway from the survival brain to the guru brain goes from being a one-lane road to a superhighway (it actually gets measurably bigger and faster). We get quicker access to our inner guru, our inner wisdom, which calms us right down if we are getting too riled up. This is what decreases our stress response to life's events. We access our inner wisdom faster. This access shifts our perspective, and we just don't sweat the small stuff. It's not that we're learning to manage stress—the stress response just does not happen.

The overall effect of this quick access to our inner wisdom is a reduction of stress hormones, which helps many bodily functions, such as blood pressure and circulation, respiratory (breathing) function, and the perception of pain and body discomfort, and lowers the risk of artery blockage, heart rhythm disturbances, and heart attack. Through the changes in the brain pathways it also modifies fear and anxiety. It also enhances immune system function. Not a bad set of outcomes for twenty minutes a day—the minimum amount needed for lasting change—of meditation practice.

This is why I chose meditation as one of the core treatments for my cancer. It really tunes up the body's functions. When diagnosed with cancer, my guru brain said, "Don't sweat it. We won't know what death is like until we get there." Dying is what it is, and there is no reason to stress out over it in advance. Meditation, gratitude, and letting go of control had cured my fear of death.

Although meditation can seem like a difficult task for most of us, starting small and building on a practice is the easiest way. Learning from recorded teaching, as I did, is cheap and easy. In teaching meditation, I found that if you start with five to ten minutes of practice twice a day, it is easier to control your busy brain. Because of this, I created my own meditation CD that guides the student on building a practice.

Another way to start is to attend a class. I often recommend this as well. Like learning any new skill, meditation takes practice on a daily basis. The skill set builds as the brain changes and the practice starts to feel natural. There may be some days when you can't stop your busy mind. Don't worry; after thirty years of practice, I still get to laugh at my thoughts, which just won't shut up!

In Buddhist philosophy, meditation is described as a way to help us decrease suffering. Suffering is described as a lack of contentment or peace. It arises when our expectations are not met by our real-world experience. Now I no longer had to suffer with the mundane aspects of my life, and I didn't have to suffer with the far less mundane issues around dying. Suffering is optional.

Meditation helps us gain a better sense of reality beyond the stories we tell ourselves about what life is supposed to be like. In essence, it offers us an enhanced awareness. It allows us to become the observer of our own stories (our Neuroimaginal world) as opposed to being controlled by them. It frees us from the small box of life that we have created and allows us to accept reality for what it is. I didn't need to be angry because fifty-two-year-olds are not supposed to die of esophageal cancer. Here I was, and so was the cancer. Anger served no purpose at all.

Meditation also helped me see that my expectations were just stories that I was telling myself about life. I became free of what life was supposed to be and able to enjoy life as it was.

We spend our entire lives making up stories about what should be and what is truth. I'm convinced that the mind just likes to entertain itself. Have you ever sat in a restaurant waiting for someone and begun to tell yourself stories about the people around you? That couple is having a fight because he's having an affair; that couple is on their first date, but it's not going well. Have you ever judged another person and created a story about what motivates him or her, only to find out that you were wrong? Our minds try to create stories to help us understand the world and fit in with our belief system. This is our Neuroimaginal world, the world we create in our heads to explain events to ourselves.

Sometimes just going within, getting quiet, and listening is where we learn the most about life, or about death. We don't need to run out and do the bucket list of seeing and doing new things. We just need to sit, listen, and learn.

This, over time, has become my philosophy of living. Pay attention to the good stuff that happens every day and enjoy what *is,* not what *should* have been or what *might* be. Enjoy every sandwich. My life is my sandwich, and I might as well savor every bite.

I thought I was doing this to find peace in my life now. This was great: less fear and anxiety and more pleasure. I didn't know that I was on the crest of the roller coaster, about to descend.

SEVEN

Do I Need to Be Locked Up?

*There are only two ways to live your life. One is
as though nothing is a miracle. The other is as
though everything is a miracle.*
—Albert Einstein

The more I meditated and practiced yoga, the more I began to experience an apparent ability to predict events, read other people, and see what others saw. This was very strange. Was this real or imagined? Was I losing my grip on reality?

I remember walking with my friend Glenn in the hills of Marin County, when his cell phone rang. I impulsively said, "Don't worry about the cream cheese." I had no idea where that came from. Glenn was the president of a large food company, and the call was to let him know that a vat of cream cheese had been sent out that might have been tainted. I had no way of knowing about the contaminated cream cheese, yet there it was—somehow I knew.

Little synchronicities and "knowings" became common, although always a surprise and always intriguing. Somehow, I was gaining insight into something that I had no access to before. It may have been an untapped part of my brain that was giving me this information or some contact with an external source of information that I did not comprehend. It was disturbing but also fascinating. My scientist mind was curious, and I began to write down these bits of intuition. I found that the more I paid attention to my intuitive hits or knowings, the more they seemed to come true. I slowly began to become comfortable with my ability to predict things. Frankly, my ego became engaged. Maybe I had super powers—the dream of every ten-year-old! I did discover that like any sense, my intuition could be cultivated by attention and greater use. This was very helpful in my career as a doctor.

It was around that time, and still several years before I was diagnosed, that I had my first experience with it being a good day to die. I had taught at a retreat for the lay public about heart disease prevention. I'd shared the stage with friends I admired, and I felt very satisfied. Kathy and I sat outside looking up at the mountain ranges surrounding Santa Barbara, breathing in the fresh air, hearing birds chirping, and holding hands. In that moment, life was complete. I had never felt that way before. I turned to Kathy and said that if I died today, it would be fine. Knowing of my capacity to see events in the future, she got very agitated and wanted me to have a full body scan (she is a doctor, after all). I let her know that I didn't feel like I was going to die, just that it would be okay if I did. I was truly at peace and satisfied with life.

As time went on, my intuitive knowing led to other experiences that I never could have imagined, to the point of truly questioning my own sanity. I began to have what could be called past-life experiences. Although I enjoyed movies and books with reincarnation themes, I was highly skeptical about their reality.

It all began on a trip to Omaha, Nebraska, where we had one of our Ornish Program for Reversing Heart Disease research sites. The yoga teacher at the program center, Susi, had said that I would enjoy meeting her friend Sandy.

Later that week, six of us from the research team were sitting on the outside patio of a small restaurant. It was a humid Nebraska night, and I could feel the moist air on my skin. During our meal, Sandy happened to walk into the restaurant.

She joined us and sat at the table across from me. As I looked at her, I had this sense that I knew her from somewhere else. It was unnerving. There was a palpable sensation that I had no understanding or experience of but could nonetheless feel in every fiber of my body. It was like the rush of adrenaline felt at the first drop of a roller coaster. But I was sitting on a deck in a health food restaurant in downtown Omaha, Nebraska. Sandy was a beautiful woman with dark brown wavy hair and deep blue eyes, but I couldn't attribute this feeling just to the typical male response to the sight of a beautiful woman. I was jittery and unsettled—much like the feeling you have after drinking way too much coffee. At the time I had no idea why I was having that reaction.

After dinner, Sandy pulled me aside and said, "You're coming with me." This surprised me, but she must have sensed something, too. I said nothing.

At a traffic light, I watched as Sandy pushed her hair back behind her right ear. In that moment I saw her not as she was today but as a different woman in an old-fashioned high-collared white dress, riding on a carriage. The woman I saw had black hair and sharp facial features.

I had seen this woman repeatedly in my dreams over the last few months but had thought nothing of it until now. Just for that second, Sandy wasn't Sandy anymore. I experienced a sense of dizziness as if dropping suddenly, like when an airplane hits an air pocket. The experience was unsettling, otherworldly, and completely real.

"Sandy, something very weird is going on."

She waited a moment and quietly said, "I know," as if it was not a surprise to her.

We drove quietly the rest of the way to the bar to meet up with our group.

We laughed and danced together. At one moment, while dancing, she put her head on my chest, and I felt like I had been hit with a two-by-four. As we talked and I looked into her eyes, I felt like I was falling into a void. I had no idea what was going on, but when I finally got to bed that night, I had chills, shakes, and surges of energy throughout my body. It wasn't a fever or an ill feeling. I later learned about kundalini experiences. These are huge flows of natural energy, much like an electrical shock wave, that pulse throughout the body as the energy floodgates open wide. Although I didn't know it at the time, I was having a kundalini experience. I called Sandy at 3:30 A.M. from my little hotel bed, sweating uncomfortably. Sandy was having a similar response. Exhausted, I finally slept for a few hours.

The next morning, on my flight home, I started to get vivid visions of London in the mid-1800s. I saw myself walking along a dirt path next to a creek with a woman named Victoria. Victoria was the woman I had seen when Sandy pushed her hair back in the car the night before. I saw us in a white three-story town house near Regent's Park, much like the house in *Mary Poppins*. I saw myself as a tall German surgeon named Richard Volkmann who was in love with Victoria. I saw the neighborhood where we took walks and the place where I went to school, and I even saw the day she died of a tubal pregnancy after a garden party (yes, I had that much detail). I had images of drinking myself to death at the age of sixty after I was unable to save her life. I thought I was having a psychotic breakdown.

On my return home from Nebraska, I had no way to explain this to Kathy. Explaining that I had recalled a past life with a beautiful woman would be hard for anyone to swallow. I could imagine Kathy asking about my trip and me responding, "Oh, it was okay. I went to the hospital, reviewed the patient records, met with the clinical team, had a nice dinner, and then went out dancing with my lover from the 1800s." This would not go down well. I couldn't yet figure out if this was just about attraction to someone else or if I was truly going crazy. I was seeing things that weren't real and feeling emotions as if they were. Was I going to end up on the street corners talking to people who lived over a hundred years ago?

This experience was so far out of the box for me that I couldn't imagine what was going on. The memories and emotions felt real, yet there was no way they could be. How could I have lived in the 1800s and be alive now? Even if that was possible, how could I remember all of this in such detail? I was truly concerned and scared about what was happening to me. Have you ever woken up from a dream that you felt was real and not been able to shake that feeling for hours after waking? Imagine that experience a hundred times stronger.

Feeling in crisis, the next morning I told my close friend Jim Billings, a psychotherapist and theologian by training, what was happening and asked him if I needed to commit myself to a psychiatric institution. His response was very clear: "No, because you can ask that question." This stopped me in my tracks. As a clinician, I knew this to be true. If I was aware that I was having these images and could separate them from "reality," I didn't need to be committed, but I certainly needed help! I was surprised when Jim said to me, "I've been waiting for this to happen." Apparently he had seen this percolating in me over many months and had expected it. Somehow this gave me a sense of peace. A close and trusted friend and therapist was telling me that I would be okay, in fact better than okay; he told me that this would be good. I couldn't believe him yet; my Neuro-imaginal box was straining to expand, but I was not quite ready.

Jim suggested I read books on spiritual emergence and past lives. Carl Jung, Stanislav Grof, and many other psychotherapists have written much about spiritual crises and awakenings over the last hundred years. I learned that many people going through difficult moments in their lives had spiritual awakenings, some of which included past lives but all of which included the awareness of the "bigness" of the universe. Those earlier explorers explained that we are just a small part of what is going on in the physical and spiritual universe, and when we become aware of this reality, we feel very, very small. We realize that we may never understand our lives and are at the mercy of many unknown forces. Although this was, for me, a very scary moment, it opened up a sense of mystery and awe I had never experienced before. My small world as a doctor, a father, and a husband was collapsing before my eyes. I was terrified and in awe at the same time.

My friend Edgar Mitchell, the Apollo astronaut, had such an experience while coming up from behind the dark side of the moon. In that moment, Edgar realized how small he was in the grand scheme of things, and even though he was a well-educated scientist, he became aware and in awe of how little he really knew about the universe and the meaning of life.

For Edgar this awe, this awakening, happened in a lunar capsule in outer space. For me it happened while riding in a Nissan in Omaha.

Slowly I began to understand that my experience was a spiritual awakening, not a psychosis. I was gaining a sense of something bigger than myself, a sense that time is not necessarily linear. This realization was very disruptive of my day-to-day life, but over many months I became increasingly comfortable with it. Not understanding the world, not having control, accepting mystery, was becoming tolerable for me.

In a religious context I was gaining a connection with God or Spirit. For me this was the beginning of letting go of control. If there was a plan, it was not mine. How could I control something that I could not truly understand?

I had always had the sense that science was not

enough to explain my life experiences and the meaning of my life, if there was a meaning to it. After these past-life experiences and as I studied further, I realized that today's science is just a collection of theories about what the world, life, and the universe might be, not what it is. We are cavemen waiting for fire. We are Newtonian physicists waiting for Einstein.

We all have inexplicable experiences of knowing. I and many other physicians have known at some deep level that a patient would live or die even though the available data might tell us otherwise. Many people I have talked with have shared dreams or intuition with close family members, knowing that something was wrong but not knowing how they knew. These experiences and synchronicities are common, yet we tend not to talk about them because we are afraid that we will be called crazy. I don't know anyone who when challenged can't reveal some such event in his or her life that could not be explained rationally.

I have read interesting research on past-life experiences. Scientists have sought out individuals, sometimes small children, who seem to have memories of lives and families that they could not have been aware of through "normal" contacts in their current lives. The late Ian Stevenson, M.D., who was at the University of

Virginia, published extensively in this area. Over forty years, Stevenson studied more than three thousand cases of past-life claims. He was able to describe and identify many past-life memories of small children, which were verified by further research. I remember the story of a small child in the Middle East who "remembered" his wife from a past life and described their life to researchers in great detail. The research teams then tracked down those families by name and found the stories to be true. There was no way a child who lived hundreds of miles away could have known those families. Stevenson also cataloged over forty cases in which unusual birthmarks on children who recalled past lives were in the same location as scars or injuries from the prior life.

His Holiness, the much-respected Dalai Lama, is supposedly the fourteenth reincarnation of past Dalai Lamas. So why couldn't I be some unknown surgeon from Germany?

I was reluctant to research my memory of Richard Volkmann, but eventually curiosity overcame my doubts. It turns out that there was a fairly well known orthopedic surgeon from Germany named Richard Volkmann who lived and died on the dates I remembered. He was a frequent visitor to London and was well known in the British medical and scientific communities. My recollection that he had a drinking problem echoed the statement of his biographers that he had ended his life "on a liquid diet." I've yet to find any information about a woman named Victoria in his life, but this may have been a relationship outside his marriage and not documented. Could I have heard the name Richard Volkmann in medical school? That's possible but highly unlikely, as he was not a historically significant figure in medicine and I am not a surgeon (at least this time around). Even if I had heard about him, I wouldn't have learned about his trips to London, the dates of his death, or his liquid diet in medical school. I remain a little skeptical still, but I have been trained to interpret data, and the data suggest to me something more than mere coincidence.

Now my life felt like a roller coaster of uncertainty. I began spontaneously experiencing glimpses of other past lives. My life as I knew it no longer existed. My worldview was changing, and life and death became even greater mysteries. I wasn't sure or comfortable with living in the here and now, yet I did passably well. At times, I barely knew what was here and now versus the past. Jim, bless him, held my hand through the process, and I was able to function fairly well. Kathy was very disturbed by all of this and didn't know what to do. Her stable physician husband, the medical director of a research institute, was *losing it!* That was not what she had signed up for, and she refused to talk about it with me: She would just shut me down every time I tried to engage her.

My world was expanding, but Kathy couldn't go there with me. This was very painful. I had to hide what was becoming a significant part of my belief system. It felt like I was living a lie. After many months and a lot of reflection, I realized that if she couldn't at least accept that for me this was real, I couldn't live with her anymore. It was the equivalent of a person who becomes religious living with an atheist who is not willing even to talk about the existence of God. But over the next few weeks, I realized that I didn't need Kathy to think like me; I just wanted her to accept me for who I was and who I was becoming. I loved her deeply and wanted to be with her, but I couldn't continue to live with her and pretend my life hadn't changed dramatically.

While we were making our bed together one morning, I said to her, "If you can't see me and accept me for who I am, I can't stay here anymore, but if you can, I want to be with you for the rest of my life." I had pondered this statement for weeks and knew that it was true.

Her eyes filled with tears, and she looked up at me and said, "I'll try." Over the next few days and weeks she asked me questions about these past-life adventures, she read Brian Weiss's book *Many Lives, Many Masters* about Weiss's experience with a patient and her past-life regression. A few months later Kathy had lunch with Brian and comfortably participated in the conversation.

My wife is truly remarkable and strong. When her feet are put into the fire, she is willing to change her perspective quickly. In many ways she sucks it up and moves on. Sometimes this is enough for me.

My past-life recollections continued to unfold. In many of them I was a physician. In one I was a physician in France during the plague who collapsed from exhaustion and lack of self-care. In another I was a young scientist in ancient Greece who cared only for science but had no life beyond his studies. And of course I was the self-centered German surgeon who could not save the woman he loved. These images would occur in my meditations, in my sleep, or in quiet moments. They were unsettling, but over a few months I began to accept and even anticipate them. The psychotic and the spiritual became the usual.

I began to see a pattern in those lives. I was often a medical professional struggling with personal issues. There was a consistent obsession with perfection, too much attention to science and not enough to humanity, overinvolvement with patients, and arrogance. In many ways, I felt like I was being given the outline for the book I wrote years later, *Finding Balance in a Medical Life.* This also led me to understand something that has become a life principle for me: It's less important to understand the source of the information than it is to understand how this information informs and directs my life today. I was not being guided to become a guru. I was being taught how to teach my colleagues through my own lives without having to reveal the source of the information. The messages of these past-life experiences were very useful.

Over the next few months I would wake up at three in the morning hearing the words *change medicine.* I was anxious about this, as the idea of changing the world of medicine seemed impossibly large. How could one person do this? Where would I start? I had no idea what it meant. I also didn't want to jeopardize my life further by leaving a job with good pay and benefits. But one can resist for only so long.

It was on a warm summer morning, while meditating in our guest room, that I was shown my death in this life. I lay emaciated, at age seventy-eight, in a bed with aluminum rails, dying of cancer, surrounded by my family. The room was hospital green. I was at peace. I saw that my work of changing medicine was finished and that I hadn't lost my family in the process (my greatest fear). It was at that moment that I agreed to take on the task of changing medicine, whatever that meant and even though I had no plan. It was also in that moment that I realized that if there was some master plan, I had no idea what it was. I could only go along as best I could. I began to let go of my need for control over the big picture.

Seeing my own death in this life and knowing that I had been here before also gave me a deep sense of the continuum of life. I knew that life did not begin or end with this one. This life was just a part of the puzzle, the mystery, and the adventure. This makes dying in this life much easier to accept. It's just part of the ride.

How can I explain all of this? I simply can't rationally.

What does the world of neuroscience tell us about experiences like mine? We may be hardwired to have them. They can occur spontaneously, without provocation, or they can occur after one has taken psychoactive drugs such as the mushrooms used in Native American ceremonies or in shamanic journeys. They can happen during prayer, starvation, depression, or sensory deprivation. The curious thing is that there are centers in our brains that create and process these experiences. These centers have been referred to as the God spot (technically the right angular gyrus and posterior right temporal region of the brain). This challenges us to consider why these centers exist at all. Do they exist to process other information and just happen to be triggered by the afore-mentioned stimuli? Did the hand of God or Spirit place them there? We may never know.

We know that when electrical currents stimulate these areas, they can trigger out-of-body experiences, experiences of communication with God, or a sense of connection with a universal energy. Although this obviously doesn't explain why we can have past-life experiences, it does suggest that somehow the God spot is a spiritual center of the brain that leads to unusual experiences of many types. At this point, all neuroscience can tell us is that they are there and don't seem to have any other discernible purpose. All I can tell you is that triggering these areas can alter your worldview. In other words, it will blow up your box!

Could my past-life experiences have been all in my mind, my Neuroimagination? It is possible that these experiences were dreamlike thoughts in a waking state, triggered by the God spot of my own brain. They seemed more real and palpable than daydreams, but this could have been the result of many years of meditation.

It is very possible that spiritual experiences are examples of our ability to tap into or gain awareness of a part of the brain of which we are not usually conscious. It is often said that we are conscious of only about 10 percent of our brain activities at any given time; what is happening out of our awareness in the other 90 percent may be what is brought to consciousness in these altered or nonwaking states. According to some researchers, those who meditate develop greater access to these unconscious parts of the brain.

Some psychiatrists and psychologists think that these experiences may be information from the collective unconscious. Carl Jung, the renowned psychiatrist, was the first to describe this. Jung talked about an unconscious space that connects all living beings. He and his students believe that we receive information from this source and respond to it even before it enters our conscious minds. With this model, I could have been tapping into this collective information pool and experiencing the images, memories, and emotions of others in the past, present, or future. Maybe this is also the source of all of our synchronicities and intuitive knowing.

I do know that these experiences felt as real as waking up in the morning, making coffee, and going to work. They were as real as any conscious conversation I have had, and I truly experienced the sense of "being there" at all levels.

What is most important to me is that these experiences filled me with questions about life's purpose and mystery. I no longer could accept the idea that I knew everything. As my worldview and life view got larger, what I knew for certain seemed to get smaller. Paradoxically, not knowing the big picture has given me a greater capacity to take risks in a world that cannot be predicted. As Helen Keller said, "Security is mostly a superstition. It does not exist in nature, nor do the children of men as a whole experience it. Avoiding danger is no safer in the long run than outright exposure. Life is either a daring adventure, or nothing." My life has been an adventure. It might have been an adventure without these visions, but they certainly added a level of depth and richness that I am grateful for.

When I started to face the reality of cancer and death, this not knowing was very comforting. Leaving this life may just mean moving on to the next one, and although this life has been extraordinary, I cannot know what awaits me in the next one. Fearing the unknown seems like a waste of time and energy. Knowing this may not be our last sandwich helps us not to regret that with each bite the sandwich slowly disappears.

EIGHT

A World of Your Own Making

Reality, what a concept!
—Robin Williams

In my old reality, you grow up, you have kids, you become a doctor, you practice medicine until you are too old and feeble to continue, you retire, and then you die. Any time any of this becomes uncomfortable, you suck it up and move on.

In my new reality, past lives are possible, death may be a stop along the way, meditation is essential, and love is the juice that fuels it all. There's room enough for many emotions, thoughts, and beliefs, and it is all part of my human experience. We can create the world we live in by shaping our own reality in our minds, and in doing so, we can reconfigure the structure and function of our brains to match our new reality.

Our reality is, to paraphrase Robin Williams, just a concept. It is a conscious and unconscious set of perceptions of the world that we believe to be true. It is based on our neurophysiologic makeup and survival physiology. It is just perception.

Perception differs from person to person because it is based on people's life experience and what they have learned about the world consciously or unconsciously. Therefore, reality differs from person to person. When I see the color blue, I don't know if you, looking at the same thing, see what I see. When I hear a statement made by someone, I don't know if you would interpret it as I would. When we go to a movie, you may have a completely different experience of it than I did, and I may never understand how you experienced it.

Men and women often struggle to understand one another. Different hormonal physiologies create different mental and emotional realities. Hormones, upbringing, and differing genetics all create different realities.

We see the world around us through the filter of our experiences, our emotions, and our physiological drives and desires: our Neuroimaginal world. We can see the world only through this lens.

This, to me, is delightful. I may never be able to know what is truly real. There will always be mystery in life. Mystery creates wonder. Not knowing gives us the freedom to explore and the curiosity to learn. The belief that we know all gives us a false sense of security and saps the urge to learn. If we knew everything, Christopher Columbus might have sat in a bar in Spain drinking wine instead of risking his life to find a new world. The world, in fact, might be a very boring place without not knowing.

> *Imagination is more important than knowledge.*
> —*Albert Einstein*

As someone who has done medical research, I know that research can answer questions only on the basis of our limited ability to think of those questions. It's an interesting game but a game nonetheless. We can identify trends that support our ideas, but that's all we can do. With this in mind, fearing death is simply fearing that which we do not understand. This fear makes no sense to me. Why should I spend whatever time I have left worrying about what might happen after I die? I am open to finding out what, if anything, lies beyond this life.

To die will be an awfully big adventure.
—*James Barrie*

Our lack of a shared reality and uncertainty can create complexity and confusion in our lives and relationships. Have you ever been in a meeting or conversation with a friend or colleague and afterward found out that you have completely different views of what happened? You were both in the same meeting, hearing the same words, witnessing the same events, yet your interpretations are completely different. Your Neuroimaginal worlds are to blame. They are just different.

Our parents and family of origin contribute significantly to the creation of this Neuroimaginal world. They take our basic brain function and add color to it in many ways. They may add a sprinkle of anxiety or a pinch of hypercaution, as my family did with me. Fortunately, my mother threw in a dollop of curiosity and my dad mixed in a heaping scoop of sweetness and humor. Families may throw in optimism, self-doubt, playfulness, adventurousness, and willingness to change or not change. These and many other ways of being are learned from our parents at a very early age. Each day we carry these learned patterns with us, consciously or unconsciously. They affect all of our life experiences, perceived choices, and relationships. If a willingness to try new things was part of your family makeup, a work meeting about change is a meeting about opportunity. If your family was all about maintaining the status quo, a work meeting about change is about threat. Same meeting, different family, different perceptions.

How has your family of origin affected your thinking on a day-to-day basis? What rules did they teach you? How do these rules affect your life? Could they be wrong?

If you enter into any conversation with your own agenda or rules, you will look for points that support your agenda and dismiss points that contradict your agenda. You don't have to do this consciously; it happens automatically. You will remember and experience the pieces you wish to hear, consciously or unconsciously. If you are optimistic, you'll see the positive aspects of the discussion; pessimists will see the negative aspects. In addition, if you had a bad morning, you are more likely to focus on the negative. If you've had a great morning, you are more likely to focus on the positive.

One deeply unconscious piece of this process is the survival brain, which surveys the world for potential danger all the time. This probably has saved your life many times. It helps you avoid getting hit by cars and falling off cliffs and tells you not to walk down dark alleys alone. The downside of this surveillance is that it perceives any and all *potential* threats as *actual* threats until proven otherwise. By nature, your survival brain overreacts. Risk and danger avoidance are a big part of this too. The survival brain can impede you from taking risks and trying new things.

We were born to survive. We are all programmed to satisfy our need for food, water, oxygen, and sleep and to reproduce. Many of our decisions and impulses are based in this survival mode. It drives many of our choices and generates much of our fear. We assume that we have choice, but often we do not. At some irrational level, we believe that if we eat right, exercise daily, and take vitamins, we won't die. Although these actions may decrease our risk of illness, they give us a false sense of safety in a world that is not in our control. We all die. We are all dying.

Death is the ultimate challenge to the survival brain. Therefore, there is a lot of unconscious vigilance about dying. Add to this the knowledge that most of us don't really know what happens after we die, and it's a double whammy, generating a greater fear of death.

The less you know about dying, the more you may fear it.

People who witness peaceful deaths or who live in societies in which death is considered a natural event have less of a fear of death. This explains why a belief in an afterlife, a belief in heaven, gives people a sense of peace around death. The unknown becomes the known through belief, not experience, and this alone can be comfort enough. This is also how people can die comfortably in the name of God. The belief in heaven or an afterlife overrides the survival brain, quelling the fear of death. Death brings glory, peace, or reward.

There is an interesting pose in yoga called the corpse pose—savasana—that consists of lying flat on the back with the palms up in a position of surrender. This simple act of lying down can be a very powerful practice of letting go of control.

I have been counseling a fellow physician who has a very significant cancer and a powerful fear of death. He has a potent religious belief in God. I've asked him to use this pose once a day for ten minutes, breathing deeply while surrendering his life to God. As his fear creeps in, he breathes deeply, releasing control. For him, for me, for all of us, we have no control over when we die; we can only relax into that thought to diminish our fears.

Interhuman connection also gives us a sense of peace. Healthy humans live to create community and fear the loss of community. It is a substantial part of our Neuroimaginal world. The chances of human survival improve when there are other supportive humans around. We protect one another against adversity, we feed one another, and we share tasks so that the group's needs are fulfilled. Community gives us a sense of safety.

This need for community can have interesting life ramifications. We create shared Neuroimaginal worlds with people who have the same interests, likes, and dislikes that we have. The need can manifest as a shared passion for a particular sports team, a type of music, or a hobby, but the real need being met is the need to bond with others. For my family, my friends, and especially my wife, the communal passion is for the San Francisco Giants. This shared enthusiasm creates a sense of community and leads to many hours of collective pain (with losses) and joy (with wins). We have a shared Neuroimaginal experience. This is the happy, enjoyable part of the Neuroimaginal world, a Neuroimaginal community based in fun.

Other, more tragic versions of these shared Neuroimaginal communities manifest as the hatred of one group of people for another (not just Giants/Dodgers or

Red Sox/Yankees). This occurs when there is a perceived threat, which may be as simple as a difference in religious or political beliefs or skin color. The community rallies together under the shared fear, which often is expressed as hatred. This enhanced sense of community is stronger than the human need for compassion and thus leads to horrific human behaviors. This is too often the sad outcome of a community-based Neuroimaginal world.

We are so quick to judge other people, yet we often can't possibly understand their perspective. We didn't grow up in the same world they did, yet we apply our rules to them. We do this as countries, coworkers, and sometimes even loved ones. This is conditional love: "I will love you if you act like the person I want you to be." If your Neuroimaginal world is just like mine, I will love you. What if we moved away from this and toward unconditionally loving others? We may not like what they do, based on our Neuroimaginal world, but we can still love them.

Unconditional love can also be made into a practice. This has been very potent for me over the last few years. Whenever someone I love is doing something I don't like, I breathe in, remembering all that that person is to me in my life. This makes the action of the moment seem small. Now, I even do this when it's not based on a situation that is bugging me. I just sit, breathing deeply, and think of the people in my life I love, a nice reminder of this tasty life in the middle of a busy day.

This practice can alter our Neuroimaginal world, which is constantly changing and can be intentionally changed. As you can imagine, if this world was created through our own life experiences and repetitive thought patterns, new experiences and the practice of new thoughts can re-create it. New experiences supply new information to our brains and actually physically enhance or diminish these nerve (neural) pathways over time. This is called neuroplasticity, the ability of the brain to change and adapt over time. Thus, our thoughts, behaviors, beliefs, actions, and practices and the beliefs of the people we surround ourselves with change our Neuroimaginations and physically change our brains.

There are amazing studies and stories of how our brains adapt through neuroplasticity to meet the demands of our world. For example, in people who were born blind, the visual cortex (the seeing part of the brain) is used for hearing and for reading Braille. It is as if they were seeing the Braille letters in their brains or hearing sight. When these areas of the brain are temporarily blocked, they no longer can read Braille.

In addition, specific areas of the brain can grow and

change with practice. The guru part of the brain (the anterior cingulate cortex) of long-term meditators is bigger than that of nonmeditators. This is due to daily use of these particular circuits and the building of the wisdom superhighway.

In animal studies, monkeys taught fine motor skills with individual fingers have growth and expansion of their sensory and motor areas for those fingers. This is the reason musicians practice. It enhances the parts of their brains needed to perform the task of playing an instrument without their even thinking about it.

Brain-changing experiences don't have to be dramatic to be effective. Every life experience changes the inner world of our brains, and just as easily, our minds and ways of thinking can modify the physiological and anatomical structure of our brains. Daily practice of yoga, meditation, and psychotherapy all change the function of our brains. Gratitude practices, meditation, prayer, and connection with others all change our Neuroimaginations and enhance our lives.

I began life in a loving family that was fearful of "others." In the Neuroimaginal world of my youth, death was tragedy, illness was terrible, and being a doctor was being a saint. I am no longer the same person I was at age five, nor am I the same person that I will be at age seventy-five (if I get there). I have moved out of the confines of my old life into a new home that is ever changing and growing.

My experiences and practices have reshaped my brain. In my Neuroimaginal world now, people are loving, fun stuff happens every day, life is an adventure, and death is no longer something to fear. Death is just what it is, something that happens to us all, at the end of what we have the opportunity to craft into a very sweet life.

So what is reality? It is the creation of our physiology, neurology, life experiences, and conscious practices. It is what our Neuroimagination tells us it is. I may never have a clue about what your reality is or what is really out there. I live in my own little world. It's a nice place; drop by sometime.

I also know that the Giants finally, after fifty-six years, won the World Series. If I have to die, that makes it even more acceptable to me. But healing my fear of death did not mean that others wouldn't suffer.

NINE

Mind Games

Brain: *An apparatus with which we think we think.*
       —Ambrose Bierce

The day after my diagnosis our son, Will (age eighteen at the time), and I were scheduled to go on a guys-only trip to his college orientation and to have fun in Los Angeles for a few days. Kathy and I decided that we wanted him to enjoy this trip and the excitement of his impending college life—at least for these few days—without worrying about my health. I still feel that this was a wise choice, but it led to four of the most difficult days of my life. I had to make a conscious attempt to control my unconscious emotions. I had to try to decrease the activity of the part of my brain that was thinking about cancer and amplify the part that was thinking about being Will's dad.

On the seven-hour drive we talked about music, base-ball, school, and life. We listened to comedy, rap, and rock and had a great time, but every so often my cancer mind would intrude, and I would get choked up and turn away to suppress my tears. I had no capacity to control the intrusions. I could only suppress my reactions. Will later told me that he knew something was wrong but didn't know what it was.

While Will and I were on the road, Kathy was trying to get our daughter, Cheryl, to come over so we could all talk when Will and I returned. She kept asking Kathy, "Why? What's going on?"

Calling me on my cell phone while I was driving with Will, Kathy told me, "I spoke to Cheryl, and she wants to know what's going on. She knows something is wrong. Would it be okay if I told her?"

"Yes," I said, holding back the tears. I wanted to be there myself to talk to Cheryl. I needed her to look into my eyes and see that her father was still there.

"So, I can tell her?" Kathy repeated.

"Yes, that would be okay," I repeated in a mechanical voice to hide my true emotions from Will.

So Cheryl found out that day without my being there to hold her and reassure her.

Will and I spent the next day with my friends Tag

and Ross and their two children, all curly hair and filled with laughter. We visited The Getty. We enjoyed the art, checked out the views, and played on the lawn. Again, I struggled not to cry as I watched other parents and their kids playing and my own eighteen-year-old playing with an adorable toddler. I imagined him as an adult with his own children, something I might never get to see. This was my first glimpse of what a future might look like without me in it. I would miss out on seeing my children get married and become parents themselves. I would never know my grandchildren. I wouldn't hear those grandchildren of mine giggle with delight as my children tickled their bellies. I would surely miss those moments.

Will and I continued on and had a great visit to Los Angeles. We toured Grauman's Chinese Theatre, checked out the movie studios, walked the Santa Monica pier, and visited some of the best basketball shoe stores in town (we both love shoes). We ate at Canter's Deli and walked Melrose Avenue. We had a blast, but my cancer mind continued to bubble up throughout all of this, dampening my mood and even, God forbid, my desire to shop for sneakers.

Arriving at the University of California, Riverside, the next day was truly exciting. We had toured the campus before, but now it was real. Will was moving into a new life and was thrilled. The campus is set against gorgeous desert hills. On this day, there were lines of cars filled with excited students and parents. We queued up for our campus orientation tour, and conversations were sparking all around. "Where are you from?" was the key topic of inquiry. I was reliving my own memories of my first day at college and feeling the anxiety and excitement of a new beginning. Many minds, many emotions, many memories all running at the same time. ·

The first orientation session was for parents and their students, but in the next session the students went off on their own. When Will left me, I began to struggle. I wanted to scream.

I knew that it was statistically unlikely that I would see my son graduate. Even more difficult to accept was the awareness that my illness would taint his first year of college in ways that I was struggling to accept. I wanted him to dive into college with all his skills, joys, and excitement, yet I knew that having me getting sicker and maybe dying seven hours away would be difficult for him. This was the hardest part for me to face, and I had no control over any of it.

Will is an amazing person: an athlete, a student, a romantic, and a truly good person. He brings laughter and thoughtfulness to any room, innocence with wisdom.

And although I worried about my illness coloring his college experience, I was comforted by the fact that I knew he had the skills, cognitive and emotional, to do well even if I were to die. I felt gratitude for the eighteen years we had enjoyed together and all the wonderful time we spent at ball games, at rock shows, and just sitting on the couch together laughing. I thought back to a punk rock show at the Fillmore when he was thrown down at my feet by slam dancers and the two of us cracked up. Most fathers don't get to do this with their sons. I knew that I had to practice gratitude for the time spent with my son and relinquish control over an unknown future. I told myself how lucky I was to have had this time, even if it was shorter than I would have hoped.

My grateful mind was repeating it: gratitude, gratitude, gratitude. All these emotions were real, present, paradoxical, and in flux. I just had to be present with them and acknowledge them all. My minds were fully engaged. Although it was difficult, I was truly alive with satisfaction, and gratitude, and grief.

It was remarkable how many thoughts were happening for me and how many stories I was telling myself: You're going to live; you're going to die; your kids will be sad; Kathy will suffer; they are strong people; they will be fine. These thoughts were spinning around in my head, and I sat there and observed them all while listening to the orientation speeches, taking notes, and reminding myself why I was there.

The next orientation day was for the students only, and I was on my own. This allowed me to focus on my pragmatic medical mind. I called my friend and colleague Mimi in San Diego, and she insisted that I come down for a PET scan. Mimi is the medical director of the Scripps Center for Integrative Medicine, and they conveniently have a PET/CT (positron emission tomography/ computed tomography) scanner. A PET/CT scanner was the next, integral, part of my cancer workup to see if the tumor had metastasized.

It felt great to be doing something about the cancer and to give all my other mind software a rest. I could stop the play that I was staging for Will and just deal with the cancer. I sat in a large, comfy chair in a softly lit room with New Age music playing while a radiated dye flowed into my veins. It felt soothing to be with my good friends at the center and to drop the facade that I had been maintaining for Will the last two days. Although I was anxious about what the test might find, I was beginning the process of being cared for by people I cared deeply about. I could get used to this. Many people have trouble being cared for. I soon learned that I am not one of those people. I have spent my life giving love and found I was perfectly comfortable receiving it.

In those few short days, I was an excited father, a proud father, someone who loves shopping and eating out, a cancer guy, a pragmatist, a loving friend, a person of sorrow, a patient, someone who allows himself to be cared for, and a professional colleague. Somehow all of those programs could run simultaneously. I was amazed that my mind could process so many thoughts and emotions simultaneously.

On the trip back home my mind began to consider how I would share the news with Will and my parents. This was not going to be easy for any of us.

TEN

The Sound of Heartbreak

There are two lasting bequests we can give our children.
One is roots. The other is wings.
—Hodding Carter Jr.

The day after Will and I returned from our trip, Kathy and I asked the kids to sit with us at an outdoor table by our pool. Towering redwood and pine trees surround our house, and the area by the pool is a place I often go to meditate. To me, it is the place where I could be calm enough to have the conversation that Kathy and I both dreaded. The kids sat down on the opposite side of the table.

"We have something to tell you that is not going to be easy to hear," I started. Cheryl held her head down, not wanting to reveal to Will that she already knew. I felt the discomfort and made a halfhearted attempt at a joke.

"No, we are not getting divorced; you're stuck with us." Nobody laughed.

"Before the trip, I was diagnosed with cancer in my esophagus."

Kathy began to tear up, but I saw her put on her medical face—supportive in light of bad news. Cheryl sat there knowingly but unable to say anything. Will looked down and asked, "Does this mean you're going to die?"

"I don't know," I said, holding back my tears and looking at this sad, sweet boy-man I loved so much. "I will have to undergo treatment and maybe surgery." I felt a need to be honest. "It's not a good type of cancer, but I will do everything that I can to stay here. To stay with you."

"I knew something was wrong the whole time we were in LA," he said.

There was not much more we could say. "We love you both, and we will go through this together." Kathy added, "We are still going to England. Dad really wants to do this trip."

I knew Kathy didn't want to go to England; she wanted me to complete my workup and start treatment right away. But to me the trip was truly important. This could be the last family trip of my life, and I wasn't going to miss it. If I was going to die, why not spend two weeks with the people I loved most?

Will asked if he could go to his room. I got up and hugged him, but he silently moved away.

Cheryl stayed and asked a few questions about treatment and if I might die.

"There is a 90 percent chance that I might die but a 10 percent chance that I will live. We won't know until we know." We smiled and hugged, and then she suggested a chemo party where people could bring me wigs and DVDs to watch. It was at that moment that I knew I had someone to laugh with about all of this. Will couldn't get there yet and Kathy was too afraid of losing me, but Cheryl could make jokes. I needed that now more than ever.

Ten minutes later, Will came up from his room and said he was going to meet his friend Dana. He could barely look my way. I felt crushed, but there was nothing I could do about it. I was powerless. I was glad that he had his friend Dana to talk to.

Cheryl and I decided to go on a hike. I needed a little moment of normality, and there is very little that I enjoy more than hiking in the hills around our town.

"Are you going to tell anyone?" she asked.

"Not yet; let's wait until we get back from England. I want to enjoy the trip and not be the 'cancer guy' yet."

We continued to talk about what all this meant: my work, our lives, what chemotherapy is like, and what other treatments might be available. Cheryl is a preschool teacher at a Montessori school and was filled with stories about the kids. "Oh, my God, Dad, this new girl is a mini-me. She's part Asian and really cute. She's so much fun to watch." She told stories about kids missing the toilet and learning how to say new words. It reminded me of how Cheryl pronounced the word *window* as a child— "windones." We never wanted to correct her. It was too cute. We laughed at how Will used to get "pachegets" (packages) in the mail and how he liked the color "lellow." These stories were all about living and learning, and that was what I needed.

Walking the dirt fire trails in the hills above our town, we noticed a rattlesnake on the side of the path, stretched out yet flicking its tongue. Rattlesnakes are not uncommon in our area, but to see one at midday in the sun is a very rare event. It must have been sick, but neither of us wanted to get too close for fear of being bitten. Cheryl and I watched it for a few minutes.

"That's powerful medicine," I said. "In the Native

American tradition the snake is the bringer of medicine, of healing."

Cheryl and I decided to take this as a good sign for my health. We were both looking for some reassurance that this would be just one of many hikes in our lives together and not the one she would need to remember or tell her children about when she thought about who her dad had been.

Will came home after a few hours with his friend Dana. He seemed calm. We stood in the kitchen and talked.

"Are you okay?" I asked, knowing that I would get a short answer.

"Yeah."

"Do you want to talk?"

"Are you going to die soon?" he asked, not wanting to hear the answer.

I felt as though I had to spin my answer in the hopeful direction. As a physician, I had done this so many times with patients that it came easily. "There is some chance that I will die from this, but even if I do, it won't be for a while. You know I know the best doctors on the planet and I will get the best treatments."

"Okay, Dad. I love you." He went down to his room,

spending most of the night talking to his friends on the phone.

In that moment, I felt his love and fear and felt the invisible thread that binds parent to child go slack for a moment. My son seemed to be practicing for my death and needed to move away from me, into life. I was powerless to make it better for him. Powerlessness was a feeling I would have to learn to get used to over the next few months.

The next impossible task was to call my parents and tell them the news. They live three thousand miles away. I had no choice.

My parents are in their early eighties and fortunately in reasonable health. They are active, they travel, and they truly enjoy their life together. In medical school we were told that the hardest life challenge to face is the death of one's child. I always presumed that this was about the loss of young children. I was fifty-three. People die at fifty-three. I figured they would be sad but not crushed. I was wrong.

"Dad, can you get Mom on the phone?"

"Sure, son. Is anything wrong?" My dad says this a lot. He tends to assume the worst first. Maybe this time he was right.

"I have something I need to tell you, so get Mom."

My mom got on the line. "Hi, what's wrong?"

"Listen, I had some trouble swallowing last week and got an endoscopy." My dad's a dentist and my mom knows quite a bit about medicine, so I could use the appropriate medical terms.

"It turns out that I have a cancer in my esophagus." I paused, waiting for a response.

My dad went to professional mode. "What does that mean? Has it spread?"

"I haven't had the full workup yet. If it's localized, I may be able to get surgery, which may be curative. If not, it will mean chemo and radiation." I was trying to sound upbeat.

I heard sniffling on the other end from my mom.

My dad tried to stay professional. "When will you know?"

"We're going to go on our trip to England. I'll finish my workup when we get back."

"You're going to England?" my mom said with dismay.

"Yes, it may be my last chance to do a family trip, and I don't want to miss it. A two-week delay won't change anything." Looking back, this was probably not the right thing to say. I heard sniffling and gasping from both my mom and my dad.

I just screwed up, I thought to myself. I shouldn't have said it might be our last family trip. But it was the truth, and I couldn't change the truth.

After another minute of forced conversation, my parents said they would call back. I got off the phone, and Kathy asked me how it had gone.

"Not good. I guess it doesn't matter what age your child is; losing them still sucks."

What my parents couldn't grasp was that I truly was okay. I was not going to England because it was going to be a last family trip; I was going to England because I wanted to have fun, I wanted to keep enjoying life regardless of cancer, and I was still fully alive.

ELEVEN

The Sickest Patients Are Sometimes the Healthiest People

Every man dies—not every man really lives.
—*William Ross Wallace*

I was on the phone for most of the day, every day, for the next two weeks. There were phone calls to family and friends, doctors' appointments, e-mails to colleagues about treatment options, and trying to figure out what to do with my work life. I was becoming the patient. Cancer life was busy.

I moved forward with our plans to go to the UK, stubbornly determined not to let cancer get in the way of the flow of life for my family and me. The experience was worth it—Will's first legal beer, fish and chips, visiting friends in London and Cambridge, the arts festival in Edinburgh, and toffee pudding, a sweet, sticky indulgence that can easily slide down an obstructed esophagus, a sweet reminder that I was still alive. I was not going to allow my illness to damage this family excursion even though every so often thoughts that this might be our last family trip would creep in. In my mind I was cataloging each event as if it would be the last, the one I would need to remember, the one that Kathy and the kids would need to remember. In my cancer mind, I was already leaving.

It took me two weeks and a lot of conversations with my physician colleagues and Kathy to realize and accept that my work life was over for the next eight months to a year, if not forever. It had taken me many years to build my career. My obsessive nature and my passion for my work had led me to an expansive—and sometimes overly expansive—career. Years of just getting by financially had left me concerned about our financial future.

The idea of cutting back or even stopping my work was threatening at a deeper level. My core belief that "I am what I do" was being challenged. Letting go of my work was a real admission that I might actually be dying.

It meant accepting that the work I loved might die with me. It meant that I was slowly disappearing.

My work life involves traveling at least half the time. On chemo and radiation, this would not be sustainable. The moment I was able to accept that my life's work might die, I had an unexpected and surprising sense of freedom. After a lifetime of being responsible, I had permission from my family and colleagues to be irresponsible. Everyone understood that my only job now was to try to recover from the disease that lived in my body, to take care of myself, and to take all the time I needed to do so. I realized that I could now stop traveling around the world and just stay home with Kathy. I had the perfect excuse to do whatever I wanted; I could pull the cancer card (now referred to by my family as the "C card"). My irresponsible, impulsive self was in full bloom. No one can refuse the C card!

I knew intuitively that the best therapy for me was to quiet down, stop being busy, meditate an hour or more daily, hike, and choose what treatments, either conventional or complementary, would maximize my healing capacity. Our bodies have an incredible capacity for self-healing. We have an intricate and complex immune system that knows what to do with cancer; in fact, all of us have abnormal, cancerlike cells that develop in our bodies regularly. The immune system recognizes and kills those cells as they appear. I knew that my job was to take care of my body with moderate exercise, lots of sleep, and good healthy food and to get my thinking brain out of the way. Meditation and time in nature became my primary treatments.

I knew that the quieter my life became and the more peace I cultivated, the greater my chances of surviving my diagnosis. I also knew that even if I did die, dying at peace would be my preference.

I contacted many colleagues and friends in the medical community to explore my other treatment options with this type of cancer. I am truly blessed to know many of the greatest hearts and minds in medicine. There was no clear choice. I had to choose the path of treatment that fit my intuition and my lifestyle in the best way possible. I could do Chinese medicine, Native American medicine, or homeopathy. I could go live in an ashram. I could go to Mexico and live on raw foods. I could be treated with chemotherapy, accepted and experimental. I could use herbs, supplements, acupuncture, and many other forms of alternative treatment. Sometimes in life, it's easier to have fewer choices.

On returning from the UK, I had to get a series of scans, biopsies, and blood work. During this workup it was discovered that I did in fact have metastasis to the lymph nodes in my neck and chest. A surgical cure was out as an option, and my chance of surviving a year dropped to 25 percent. The chance of surviving five years dropped to less than 10 percent. I embarked on an eight-month plan of chemotherapy, radiation, acupuncture, and supplement therapy along with deepening my meditation practice. I decided to keep my spirit and mood alive through music, movies, hiking, and spending time with the people I loved most.

Through all of this, laughter and tears came easily, and my lack of anxiety and fear continued to surprise me. I felt fully alive, joy became more expansive, and sorrow was deeper. My emotions flowed freely, unobstructed by my busy thinking, planning mind. I had no use for that part of me; that part of me was on hold for now, maybe forever.

I had no desire or will to fight cancer. I just wanted to be with cancer. I realized that the desire to fight cancer through extreme methods comes from a fear of dying. As I had no fear, I had no fight. This attitude upset Kathy and pissed off my medical friends. They all had elaborate plans for how I could beat the cancer. "If I had cancer, this is what I would do" was the message, which I heard and politely declined.

Fortunately, I had the opportunity to talk with Bernie Siegel, a cancer surgeon and the author of *Love, Medicine and Miracles,* early in my treatment process. Bernie understood that diving into quiet, nature, and music was a valid treatment plan along with chemo, radiation, acupuncture, and supplements. To him, I was not giving in to cancer; I was quietly being with my cancer, and that was fine.

I also knew that the more fear and anxiety I had, the higher my stress hormone levels would be. High stress hormones wear down the immune system's function over time, giving cancer a better chance to grow. Fear promotes cancer growth; calm decreases it. My mode of being became "get quiet, enjoy life, and let my body do what it knows how to do—cure cancer."

I now understand why our societal attitude toward cancer is to fight it and beat it: It is driven by a fear of dying. Look at the titles of some popular books on dealing with cancer:

Anticancer
Beating Cancer with Nutrition
The Cancer-Fighting Kitchen
Foods to Fight Cancer
A Cancer Battle Plan

How to Fight Cancer & Win
Winning the Battle against Prostate Cancer

The content of these books can be very useful, but the titles are fear-driven and anxiety-provoking. The attitude "I'm going to beat this thing" makes everyone who dies a loser. Death is a fight that no one can win.

While I was in treatment for my cancer, I was filled with gratitude for the people, things, memories, emotions, and events I had already experienced in my life. I had cultivated this attitude over many years, and it was of critical importance to my feeling fully alive in that moment. I knew, deep within my heart, that one more great meal, one more great rock show, or one more night of snuggling with Kathy would not make my life any better than it already was.

I also knew that I could die at any time and that I would have no control over the final moments of my life. Instead of worrying about when I might die and adding anxiety to each day I had left, I decided to enjoy the time I had with good music, good food, lots of love, and the quiet time that my soul and immune system needed.

I also had a strong sense that there was something else out there that I couldn't understand: what happens when we die. If I couldn't understand it, why fear it? I had a profound feeling that this life is not all there is. This, too, was liberating. Here I was dying, yet I felt fully free, fully alive. Being fully alive, I discovered, has nothing to do with the presence or absence of disease.

Our current medical system would have us believe that being fully alive is being without disease, yet we all know that it is impossible to avoid disease and that everyone will die at some point. In simple terms, our current medical system is set up to fight the inevitable—a losing battle for sure. It would have us believe that we are all losers.

One of Kathy's patients, a woman in her mid-sixties, had been diagnosed with breast cancer eighteen years before her visit to the clinic. At that time she was a new grandmother of a baby boy and made a deal with God that if she could see him graduate from high school, she would be ready to go at that moment. The woman came to see Kathy with a large lump on her head, which turned out to be a recurrence of her tumor. She knew that God was calling her back, and she was ready to go. She was happy to have had the last eighteen years to be with her grandson and didn't need any more. After all, a deal is a deal. Her daughters met with Kathy and insisted that their mother get every treatment possible to fight this cancer. They began to fight with Kathy and their mother, insisting that everything and anything be done to postpone her death. They were simply afraid of losing their mother. Kathy wisely asked the daughters to leave the room, sat with the mother, and heard her story. Kathy then went on to support the mother's decision not to be treated even though this upset the daughters greatly.

A few months later, the woman died peacefully. Soon after her death, Kathy received a letter from the daughters thanking her for supporting their mother's wishes. They had transcended their fears of losing their mother by watching her die a happy and peaceful woman, fully alive in her own death. This woman was vital, joyful, unafraid, and at peace with her God.

When I teach my students about gaining joy in their work, I have them write down the parts of their days that give them pleasure or excitement. I have them reflect on what energizes them and the coworkers they love. I ask them to work on increasing those aspects of their work so that they are spending more time doing what they love with people they care about. Over time, this shifts their perception of work, gives them a greater sense of choice and control, and makes each day more meaningful. It brings vitality to their workplace and to their lives.

Can you imagine a health care system in which the main goal is to enhance peace, vitality, and the joy of living, a system that views dying as a natural process instead of something to be feared and avoided? In many other cultures, death is looked upon as a natural event and peaceful deaths are celebrations of the person's life, not steeped in tragedy. In these cultures there are celebrations, wakes, and sweet reminiscences of people's lives; gratitude for having been with them; and the joy of knowing that they are with God. Yes, they are missed, but they are celebrated and loved. What if our health care system could be based on this awareness instead of the disease-avoidant system that we have today?

My belief in this paradigm of care led to some intense and exciting discussions with my friend Barbara, who works at the National Institutes of Health (NIH). I told her about Kathy's patient with breast cancer and how she lived and died so well. We laughed about an institute of health that spends billions of dollars annually studying disease but spends virtually nothing studying what makes people happy and vital. The National Institutes of *Health* doesn't really study health at all; it studies disease. Perhaps the NIH should be called the National Institute of Avoiding the Inevitable.

What if we could create a section of the NIH that studied health? Barbara and I realized that we were in a position to do this together with all our friends and colleagues worldwide. Over the next few months we arranged a series of meetings and conference calls, bringing together a fabulous small think tank of health leaders.

Then, within a few weeks of each other, Barbara and I were both diagnosed with metastatic cancer. This seemed to be beyond coincidence, and we were able to laugh together about the irony that is life. You may find it odd that two people facing their own mortality could laugh, but as Barbara said, we were still us, just us with cancer. We were committed to making a difference, and cancer was simply another obstacle to manage in our quest to do inspired work.

Barbara and I were living life on life's terms. We were more than the sum of our blood counts and the size of our medical charts. Cancer could not stop us, and we refused to let it define us. We knew we might die sooner rather than later, but isn't that true for all of us? Do we stop playing, creating, and loving because it could all be over tomorrow? Or do we continue to strive to make meaning out of each moment and opportunity out of each obstacle? We became like Kathy's patient: fully alive with cancer. But that didn't mean I had any control of where I was going.

TWELVE

Where No Me Has Gone Before

Living involves tearing up one rough draft after another.
—Author unknown

Cancer was now a dominant presence in my life, and I entered a world that was completely unknown to me. In my precancer world I was in charge of my life. Now there was no plan and no map to follow.

One of Kathy's coworkers survived lymphoma and lived to have a baby after her cancer. She hugged me one day and whispered in my ear, "It never goes away." I was now living in a world that only other people with cancer could understand. It is a world where life is precious yet fleeting, where the usual and normal are on hold, and where even my family couldn't possibly understand what I was going through.

I knew that I was entering the valley of the shadow of death, and I was going to look at mortality, pain, and suffering face-to-face. Part of me has a deep warrior spirit that can push forward into anything. This part of me was ready to face the suffering before me. It was ready to go into battle and emerge victorious. I had been studying Native American healing for many years and had even done work in that area. I had learned some of the shaman's tools by working with and studying with friends who taught in this area of healing.

In the Native tradition, shamans often go through a period of suffering that brings them to the point of near death. At a deep level, I knew that this was my time to suffer. I also knew that pain and suffering bring the opportunity for great transformation. I was ready to survive and hoped that I would come out of this a stronger person for the experience. I had what I believed was good training from my friends, and I was surrounded and supported by the people in my life. I was ready.

I had learned that I had many parts of myself. I have learned this way of thinking from many great psychotherapists and have taught it to other doctors. One particularly helpful way of working with the many voices competing for our attention in our heads is called psychosynthesis, a process created in the 1920s by the Italian psychiatrist Roberto Assagioli. He describes our inner parts as "subpersonalities"—in essence, our inner team.

As we are exposed to more and more life circumstances and people, we modify our behaviors to fit the environments in which we live. We create a work self, a student self, a parent self, and a caregiver self. These become some of our subpersonalities—parts of ourselves that allow us to fit into our environment and our community. We do this so that the group will not ostracize us. This is how many of our subpersonalities develop, out of a need to survive and fit in.

Think of the inner parts of yourself, those parts which develop in response to the demands of your life— your work self, your play self—different from each other in many ways yet still part of the complete you. If you spend enough time evaluating yourself this way, you will see that you have many inner selves or subpersonalities.

With my treatment pending, I was now ready to use my subpersonalities to help me get through this difficult time. Knowing that I had this capacity gave me a significant sense of peace. I knew that I could deal with pain, nausea, and even wasting away into death. I came up with a plan. My inner playful self was going to go to as many rock shows as I could while parking my inner cancer guy to the side. I would get in touch with my inner pragmatist, who would help me cancel my work life and deal with the financial ramifications of my illness, attending to disability coverage and school loans for Will. While my inner pragmatist was doing this, my inner doctor, along with his trusty colleague Kathy, was going to explore the best treatment options and come up with a plan that involved mainstream and alternative treatments for my cancer. And during this process, I was going to develop a new subpersonality: my inner patient. I could use the part of me that could be cared for and allow it to grow. A challenge would be to balance this with my inner doctor, who had dominated for so many years.

My inner shaman was also ready for this journey, and he had help: My loving heart would draw to me the people I needed, my inner guardian would create protective walls to assure needed rest, and my inner guru would keep me connected to Spirit. I had a whole team inside waiting to help. I was good to go.

I also had to relearn how to manage my relationships. After I told my parents about my diagnosis, they called me every other day. I swear they just wanted to know I was still alive. I began to call them preemptively every time I had a good day: my inner pragmatist and inner loving son working together. This was the best way to manage their fears. I would remind them consistently that I was not only alive but enjoying myself: "I just went on a hike." "I went to a great concert last night." Each time they were surprised and delighted. I was hoping that they would see that even if I was dying, I was still living fully and enjoying every moment. At some level, I was hoping to transform their views of death. This was my way of caring for them, but this too would change.

My cousin was getting married in mid-September, and this was a perfect reason for my parents to come visit us. I felt like I would need to put on a "Lee's doing fine" show. Two days before they were to arrive, I was doing volunteer work at the Saint Vincent de Paul Society, helping to develop a lifestyle-based recovery program for homeless drug addicts. Sitting in the crowded board-room, I began to experience a pain in my left lower chest. It was subtle at first, so I thought nothing of it and continued the meeting.

On my drive home the pain increased, and I thought about going to the hospital. However, it was not bad enough to warrant an ER visit yet.

When I got home, Will and I watched the comedy *Elf* with Will Ferrell, and as I laughed, the pain got much worse. I knew at that point that the pain was coming from my lung lining or chest wall and not my heart, so I decided to wait it out.

Kathy came home. "Are you sure you don't want to go to the hospital?" she asked.

Stubbornly, my inner horse's ass said, "Let's just see if it gets worse."

It did, to the point where an hour later I could barely get off the couch. "Can you and Will take me to the hospital now? Help me get up; I can't move."

Will looked scared for the first time since my diagnosis. My playacting the role of the strong cancer guy was crumbling before his young eyes. I think this was the first time he realized that I might actually die, and it clearly terrified him.

He helped me to the car and to the emergency room with Kathy. Every bump and every turn caused pain. Fortunately, the hospital was close to our house.

The pain was so severe that I couldn't even sit down to give the registration person my information for admission. I was sweating, short of breath, and unable to focus. They rushed me into the back and hooked me up to monitors and an IV. I had never been on this side of the ER before; I had never been the one in the stretcher. It felt odd, but I was relieved to be there—the pain was intense.

My inner doctor heard, "Fifty-two-year-old white male with adenocarcinoma of the esophagus complaining of progressive pleuritic chest pain and shortness of breath which started about five hours ago and has worsened since. He has no history of cardiac disease, no diabetes, no past pulmonary disease except mild allergic asthma. He had eaten about two hours ago. He is diaphoretic. His EKG is normal, he is oxygenating well on a two-liter nasal cannula. His vitals are stable." This is medical lingo for "This dude is sick. He's got cancer, and I bet he has a clot in his lungs. That's why he can't breathe. Fortunately, he's not ready to die yet."

By then, Kathy and I were convinced that I had a pulmonary embolus (PE), a blood clot to the lungs that stops that area of the lung from working.

After hours of pain, one quick injection of Dilaudid (a strong narcotic) sent a rapid wave of sweet relief flushing through my body like a soothing warm blanket. Within moments, I was nearly pain-free. This stuff is good! I can see why people become addicted to pain medication.

I had a test called a spiral CT scan that showed that I did have a blood clot in the far end of my lower left lung. That was why I was in so much pain: The clot was killing my lung lining where all the nerve endings are.

The emergency room team wanted to admit me to

give me blood thinner injections every twelve hours and to watch me to make sure I wasn't going to crash.

I needed some control over the situation, so my inner stubborn doctor announced, "I can give myself the necessary injections; I don't need to be in the hospital just to get injected every twelve hours. I am more likely to get an infection here. If I'm going to be miserable, I'd rather be miserable at home." (My inner horse's ass and my inner stubborn doctor are on very good terms.)

Kathy somewhat reluctantly agreed. I was getting enough oxygen, and I was stable. After a brief call to my oncologist, he reluctantly agreed to release me.

That night I took Dilaudid for the pain, but the Dilaudid that I could use at home was at a lower dose than I could get via IV at the hospital, and my pain was not well controlled. I tried to read but couldn't. I finally just surrendered to the severe pain. I sat there breathing, meditating, and simply trying to make it through the night. My inner guru helped me by reminding me that this was just a transient event and the pain would be gone in a few days.

My parents came the next day for my cousin's wedding. Kathy picked them up and on the way to the house told them what had happened. When they saw me, they were shocked. I was doped up, in pain, and struggling to breathe; I was the dying son they feared seeing. I knew that inside they were falling apart, but they tried to put on a good face.

"You're not going to the wedding, are you?" they asked.

"Yes, I am going. Kathy can drive, and I'll drug myself up." My inner survivor was not giving up on life.

We all sat outside, and for the first time I can remember, my father just held my hand without saying anything—no words of encouragement, no words of wisdom (as my brother and I call his speeches about life). He had always been afraid to do this, but I was suffering and he was suffering too. I remembered my father holding me as a small child, and for just a moment, I was that child being held and comforted by his daddy.

I knew that my journey had just begun and I would be facing my deepest fears and wounds over the next few months. I would need to go to places that were psychologically and spiritually uncomfortable. I would be learning a lot through pain and physical suffering, and I was ready, if anxious, to do the hard work of looking at my life, seeing myself suffer, and watching the people I loved suffer with me. I knew that this would bring out the worst in me and also the best.

I had seen this over and over again in my heart

patients approaching death—they had to face the prob-lematic sides of their lives and their personalities. They had to speak the unspeakable; they had to say what had not yet been said. They had to complete the complex puzzle of life that they had created. In doing so, they in-evitably came out happier, livelier, and, if needed, more ready to die. I was willing and prepared to dive into this world of uncertainty and face myself.

THIRTEEN

Digging in the Dark

Do you want to be good or do you want to be whole?
—*Carl Jung*

As I began treatment and learned to deal with nausea and pain, I also began a deep process of introspection. Every time in my life I had investigated the inner pain and faced parts of myself that made me uncomfortable, I would come out on the other side feeling cleansed. What better time to do this inner work than when I was going through chemotherapy?

As a student of many great teachers and as a teacher myself, I had many techniques that I could use to go within. One of my favorites is Shamanic Breathwork, which had been taught to me by my friends Nita Gage and Linda Star Wolf. This process uses rapid breathing similar to what is called pranayama in yoga, combined with music or drumming to bring a person into a trance-like state. This technique seems to trigger the God spot in the brain. In this breathwork, people have visions and see colors and animals, and often vivid, dreamlike stories play out in their minds. In these states people get a sense of receiving messages, maybe from their higher minds, maybe from the collective unconscious as Carl Jung called it, or maybe from God. Often one loses a sense of time and place.

A brief word of caution: These experiences can be very powerful. Sometimes they are very pleasurable, but they can be extremely difficult. As with any powerful psychospiritual practice, I strongly encourage students to work with an experienced guide.

In the Native American tradition, these experiences are interpreted as a connection with Spirit in which healing can take place. As I was certainly looking for healing from all sources, this was an inexpensive and powerful technique to turn to. I began to use my journey techniques fairly regularly. In these journeys, I would put on music (*The Spiral* by Soulfood) that is designed to move you through the energy centers of your body (chakras in yogic language) and allow your body energy to flow. I would pay attention to the images and emotions that would arise for me and see if they had any meaning in my life. In other journey sessions, I would do the rapid breathing used in Shamanic Breathwork with the music, always while being watched by another person.

During one such journey, I had an image of my cancer cells as black moths in my chest, and asked the moths what they were there for. They told me that they were holding my anger so that it would not kill me. I came to see that I was still struggling with how to deal with anger and with how to forgive.

I sat with this thought for some time. I realized that for many years, I had been holding a significant level of anger toward Harriet, a consultant whom I had worked with in the distant past. She had done some very disruptive things, both personally and financially, and held great financial fears. This led her to do some distrustful things and to say some very threatening things to me. She believed that in some way I was trying to hurt her. I had never had anyone act that way with me before, and it shook my beliefs about humanity, and I realized that I was still holding this unprocessed anger.

In my Neuroimaginal world at that time, I believed that everybody eventually does the right thing. People should act with compassion toward one another. Believe it or not, dealing with this person's behaviors was harder for me than dealing with the cancer. Cancer is in my

Neuroimaginal world—it just happens—but betrayal and harassment just don't happen to good people.

I realized that this anger, which was still waking me up at night and infiltrating my days, was doing me harm. I would go so far as to say that it may have triggered my cancer or diminished my immune system's capacity to deal with the cancer when it arose.

I knew then that I needed to address this anger, not avoid it. I needed to dive into it in order to transcend it. First I did this through journeywork in which I would be with the cancer cells and my anger. This allowed me to understand how big the anger was. It was overwhelming because it was not in my control.

I started by using fairly violent imagery to manage the anger. I needed some way to vent it. Somehow I needed control over it. First I would see myself shooting this person in the chest and pushing her out to sea on a raft. Although that gave me a little sense of control and revenge, it was not effective in eliminating the anger; this technique was still based in violence and actually amplified my rage. I then moved to putting her on a raft and pushing her out to sea while waving goodbye to her at the shoreline, but deep inside I still wanted to shoot her. Clearly, the anger was still there. This was not working.

My friend Marty Rossman, an expert in visualization,

suggested that I personify the anger, in essence find a character that could represent the anger. I visualized a sleazy guy with the head of a squid. Marty then told me to let the squid head blow huge bubbles and release them into the atmosphere. Though this may sound silly, it had a profound effect, lightening my anger and making it laughable, allowing a great release.

Soon after, in a meditation, I felt my chest break open, and all the black moths flew out and became black angels. I saw my anger and cancer release. It sounds quite New Agey to my inner doctor, but this simple technique worked. You can try this imagery yourself: If you are mad at someone, turn that person into a character and have him or her blow bubbles into the air. Sounds comical, but there is great transformation and healing when anger is allowed to become laughter.

On a spring day when I could barely get out of bed, I had a session with my friend Linda Star Wolf, a shamanic teacher and founder of the Shamanic Breathwork Process. I lay on the couch, bundled up in blankets and wearing my wool hat even though it was a warm spring day—chemotherapy had left me with little capacity to generate heat. Star Wolf put on music for the journey and sat next to me.

I dropped first into a meditative state and then into

a trancelike state, disconnected from my body, as if I were dreaming. I saw myself as a five-year-old telling a five-year-old Harriet that I meant her no harm because I wanted her to realize that she was safe. This was my first instance of compassion toward her. I watched her throw up her five-year-old arms and walk away. I knew in that moment that no solution could be found by talking things over. Whatever I would say to her, she could not or would not hear it. At the end of my journey, I clearly heard the words "You don't have to die for her this time." I had no idea what that meant.

While I was journeying, so was Star Wolf. She lay in a lounge chair next to me, also in a trancelike state, having her own journey parallel to mine. She didn't know much about Harriet but told me she had seen the two of us as priests in another life. Harriet, a man in this past life, was older and had high ambitions in the church to become bishop. I was his young student who loved the church, children, gardening, and teaching. I was perfectly content to do those things without any need to rise in the church community. Star Wolf told me she saw that over many years I had become beloved by the church and eventually was made a bishop. This apparently infuriated Harriet, who poisoned me.

Perhaps that's what "You don't have to die for her this

time" meant. I realized that somewhere in my unconscious mind I thought that if I died of my cancer, maybe
Harriet would recognize the error of her ways. The truth
was that I was not responsible for her actions. She would
do whatever she was going to do, and I would not be the
martyr. If she continued her life in delusion, it was the
choice of her soul, not mine.

Was this shared journey imagined? When two people share the same images in a journey, as they often do,
is this an interpersonal energetic experience, an experience of being in the collective unconscious at the same
time, or an experience directed by God? All that I know
is that it helped me let go of a need to change Harriet and
helped me to move past my anger. I was beginning to
forgive her, and in doing so I was able to move forward
with my life. Another person might say that she was now
in God's hands, not mine. I was free.

Even after this experience I occasionally would feel
anger toward Harriet, especially when I didn't feel well
physically. I was disturbed that she continued to threaten
and harass me while I was dealing with cancer; it seemed
unfair and cruel. During a chemotherapy break months
later, I was lying on a beach and realized I needed guid-
ance in dealing with my anger. I felt that I needed the help
of a higher power; I was powerless to manage it myself. I

asked God, "How can I be more Christ-like in my anger toward Harriet?" Even as someone who was raised in a Jewish tradition, I admired the work and teachings of Jesus. There, on the beach, an answer came to me: Even though I couldn't condone her behaviors, I could generate compassion for her. I should let Harriet know that I was sorry that she was suffering regardless of the reason she was suffering. I wrote her a letter saying just that. Having compassion for her helped me manage my anger.

I try to see myself in the other person's shoes and mind and try to see why people feel the way they do. It may not resolve the issues at hand and I may not approve of the choices the offender has made, but I may be able to generate compassion toward that person. Harriet felt rejected by me, and in feeling that way she reacted in ways that were destructive and vengeful. I could at least understand this, as there have been times in my life when I have dealt with rejection and wanted to be vengeful even if I didn't act it out.

A core reason why we struggle to forgive is that we believe that by forgiving we are letting the offender off the hook. This is not true. Fred Luskin of Stanford University suggests that we "forgive and remember," not forgive and forget. Forgive and move on with your life, remembering not to repeat the same mistake.

I had a choice to stay angry or not, and when it came down to staying angry and threatening my physical and psychological health, I chose to let go. I do not forget Harriet's actions and will be diligent not to find myself in a similar circumstance again. I forgave and remembered. Forgiving is empowering. We gain control of our thoughts and feelings.

Beyond forgiving others, we often struggle with forgiving ourselves. Most of us have parts of ourselves that we are not proud of. My angry squid head is one of those. I was not comfortable thinking of myself as an angry guy, but I do get angry sometimes. This is one of the many shadow sides of my personality: the parts of us that we are ashamed of or embarrassed by, the parts of us we wish we didn't have. I no longer deny them; they are part of me.

Because most of us would rather be Glinda the Good Witch and not the Wicked Witch of the West, we all really work hard at suppressing the shadow parts of ourselves. Good luck with that! The shadowy parts of our character will still show up when we least desire them and when we most need to learn from them.

Carl Jung used the term *shadow* to name the parts of ourselves that we do not want to acknowledge and often disown. Our shadow personality parts are often unconscious and arise without our awareness or control. There was a part of my personality that I called my inner Black Cape. He was very powerful but often dangerous. This part of me would yell and scream at the kids when I was tired, overwhelmed, or frustrated in a way that truly felt out of control. This was not just being a firm dad; it was tyrannical and over the top. I hated myself when I did this. My inner good dad did not like it when the inner Black Cape showed up, and I never knew when he would appear.

I could not understand this shadow part of me until I understood why it was there, accepted it, and was able to use and appreciate it as part of my inner team. I realized that the Black Cape protected me by separating me from others when I was overwhelmed but that I could meet this need without lashing out at people I loved. I was able to harness the energy of the Black Cape in productive ways to be forceful but not hurtful. He has been a very useful ally in my work life and home life and an enormous source of energy.

If you want to explore this area, make a list of the parts of your inner self that you are afraid of or embarrassed by. Then try to identify the purposes they serve. In doing so, you may see that there are other, less harmful ways of getting those needs met.

The most important misconception about the shadow side of ourselves is that it is all negative, bad, wrong, evil, and to be avoided at all costs. One need only look at wars started in the name of religion to know this. Most religions are based on the concept of loving others, yet the shadow nature of humans within religions allows us to kill each other to defend our religious beliefs. Focusing on being good and avoiding evil without healing the shadowy side is often what keeps us locked in our own negative reactions and feelings of hatred and mistrust. Once we can accept those parts of ourselves, we can work with them. Until we accept those parts, we are stuck.

Our shadow side is far more liberating and much less disturbing than any of us can imagine. Artists of all genres learn to embrace and express their shadow through their work, and this resonates with us all. Many of the greatest works of art have arisen after profound depression, anger, or loss. When Duke Ellington was refused a room in the hotel he was to play at, the next day he said, "I merely took the energy it takes to pout and wrote some blues." He took the angry, dark Duke and made it into the creative Duke. This is truly the power to use dark energy to its fullest.

To get to our passion and purpose we must be willing to shine the light of awareness on the shadow parts of ourselves. If we cannot admit it when we are angry, the anger will leak out in ways beyond our control and we will remain stuck in the anger. By acknowledging anger, we are able to make conscious choices about how and when we express that anger. Just as we have seen that we can transcend fear, we can transcend anger. All of our "negative" emotions are part of our humanity. If we can forgive ourselves for our humanity, we can forgive others for theirs.

FOURTEEN

Me, Myself, and I

We are not human beings having a spiritual experience.
We are spiritual beings having a human experience.
—Teilhard de Chardin

In my journey over the last few years and during my con-
valescence, the question of who I really am arose power-
fully and profoundly. Am I the physical being I see in
the mirror each morning? Am I a soul living in this body
that will move from body to body over many lifetimes?
Is this life just an illusion?

Defining the self by bodily limits comes into question
in a very simple experiment often performed in Psych
101 classes around the country. A person is asked to sit
at a table with one hand above the table and one hand
below it. On the table is a rubber hand placed where the

person's real hand would have been. The subject's hand under the table is stroked with a feather while the rubber hand is being stroked. The subjects are confused about which hand is real. They feel the tickle of the feather in the rubber hand and sometimes try to pull it away; they perceive the rubber hand as the real hand. When the fingers of the rubber hand are bent backward, these individuals fear pain and withdraw the real hand.

The substitution in the subject's mind of the rubber hand for the real hand occurs because the brain creates an internal imaginary construct of what the body is and where its boundaries lie. To keep us from hurting ourselves, the brain needs to know where the body is at all times, and to do this it relies especially on the senses of touch and vision. You need to know how far to extend your arm or withdraw it in any task or emergency, but this construct, created by the brain, can be fooled by a rubber hand. Our definition of the self can get re-created rapidly by the brain, so that even the brain doesn't know who we are all the time. How can we define ourselves by our physical bodies when this definition is flexible even to our own brains?

In addition, our bodies change over time. Our cells constantly are being replaced as new cells grow and old cells die off; none of the cells in your body are exactly the same cells they were a few years ago. You can tell this by looking at an old photograph of yourself. You look different now than you did when you were younger, yet you would say that you are still you. We change, we grow, we gain weight, we lose weight, we get injured, we heal. Our bodies are in flux. Clearly, the body alone can't define the self.

Can we define ourselves by our thoughts and emotions? Ask yourself if you think about and see the world the same way you did twenty years ago. Have your perceptions changed? Have your beliefs changed? Have your motivations changed? Has your knowledge changed? Your thoughts, beliefs, and emotions change from moment to moment, year to year, and decade to decade, yet you are still you. We can't therefore say that the true self is defined by our thoughts, beliefs, or emotions.

I love the following exercise. Close your eyes and say the following to yourself, repeating each statement three times:

I have a body, but I am not my body.
I have feelings, but I am not my feelings.
I have desires, but I am not my desires.
I have thoughts, but I am not my thoughts.
I am the self, the center of consciousness.

When I am too wrapped up in a thought, an emotion, or a desire, I do this for about a minute, and it helps distance me from the thought or emotion. During my radiation, I often repeat, "I have pain, but I am not my pain." It is a simple yet effective way of lessening any experience of pain.

There must be a broader definition of the self that transcends the body, emotions, and thoughts. I like to think of this as the spiritual self, the transpersonal self (in psychological language), or the one-self—a self somehow beyond the physical and beyond the body or mind. This one-self is connected to our sense of spirituality, our sense of connection with others and the universe as a whole. It is to some degree selfless. You might get a sense of the one-self while walking in nature, listening to music, praying, or meditating. In that moment you lose your mundane definition of your self. You may experience this as a connection with a higher power. You may even have a sense of this one-self when feeling love toward another or holding your child in your arms. The usual boundaries drop away, and for a moment you become one or, as Bob Marley sang, one love, one heart.

I believe that we evolve naturally toward this one-self if we allow it to happen. We begin our lives vulnerable and depend on our parents to feed us, clean us, and comfort us. When we need these things, we cry to get our needs met. Survival is our primary concern; we are always surveying for danger and always seeking safety as we age.

In our early childhood we are also social beings. We learn that when we smile, our parents smile. This gives us a sense of protection and safety. Soon we learn to expand this interaction to others, and our community grows. We learn to adopt behaviors that we see in others, allowing us to fit in and feel safe within our community. This gives us a greater sense of safety and enhances our likelihood of survival.

At some time in your life, you begin to realize that you are not made up of just the component parts of your personality; you realize that you are not satisfied with the life that was prescribed for you by family and community. You realize that something else is needed to satisfy your soul; your one-self is calling out to you for something more, something vague, something unknown, something different. You wake up to the feeling that this life may not be enough.

I believe that this restlessness, this pressure to change, moves us to evolve naturally toward this one-self if we allow it. Our human capacity to change and grow over time opens a new door of possibility: a more fluid definition of the self. Like a tree that can bend with the wind, we become more able to deal with life's changes as they arise. As you continue to push and grow, you have more one-self or selfless experiences, connections with nature, with God, with a sense of spirituality, with unconditional love, compassion, and service; you can begin to move beyond simple survival. You are no longer attached to the you of the moment. You become open to all possibilities. For me, it is this one-self that is not identified with cancer, pain, or fear. Cancer is just a physical event of the moment—it just is what it is.

In cancer treatment my physical health was terrible. I was in pain, was not sleeping well, and had little energy. My mind drifted in and out of various emotions: depression, exhaustion, anger, and at times peacefulness. My one-self, which seemed to be above my mind and able to observe it comfortably, was fine throughout the treatment, as it could experience the pain and suffering as separate from itself. It was flexible and open to whatever I was experiencing. Pain and suffering were just events of the moment, not the definition of who I was. I would survive the pain and live or I would die, but the pain and suffering would not go on forever. This gave me a sense of peace during extreme physical pain.

There was, in fact, one morning when I woke up and

had no desire to get out of bed, no desire to watch TV or read, no desire to eat, and frankly, no will to live or die. I was not depressed or fearful. I just lay there in my comfortable bed without a need to do anything. I was in a state of peace: the one-self embodied. This new sensation felt curious and interesting but not disturbing. Maybe this is what it feels like to be dying. I stayed in this state for three full days, eating little and doing nothing. There is a term in the yogic tradition called samadhi, a sense of connection with all. I believe I was in a state of samadhi at that moment.

On the third night, Kathy called our neighbors Chris and Brian. Chris was dying of cancer, and Kathy wanted to bring them food. Brian told Kathy that Chris had died that day. After she hung up the phone, she came to me, crying that I couldn't leave her. In that moment, my conscious mind decided that I could come back. I could have the will to stay alive for Kathy. I needed to drop out of this state of transcendent peace and reconnect with the pain and suffering of being in my body. This was not an attractive idea, but I was driven by the need to support the person I love most in the world. My wife needed her husband back. I got out of bed. I was back with the living.

FIFTEEN

Pennies from Heaven

God is a concept by which we measure our pain.
—*John Lennon*

In my life, I have experienced certain events that don't lend themselves to scientific explanation. During my struggles with Harriet, I asked God or Spirit, "Have I messed up somehow?" The next day, getting into my car, I found a penny on the ground. On the seat of my car was another penny. I found a few more pennies in odd places that day. No big deal. Coincidence.

That night I went to bed and tossed a pillow on the floor next to the bed. In the morning there was a penny sitting on the center of the pillow. I looked up and laughed, remembering the expression "pennies from heaven." Over the next few weeks, I found pennies everywhere I looked. I had pockets filled with pennies!

I realized that God or Spirit has a sense of humor—it appeared to be a funny message that all was well. It is easy to think that my increased awareness of pennies had me seeing pennies that I otherwise might have missed. I imagine that there are many pennies I walk past each day that I do not see. The number of pennies seemed outrageous—about ten per day for months! I certainly could not explain the penny on the pillow. I asked Kathy if she had put it there, and she gave me an incredulous look.

In my youth, I believed that God was just a story told to kids. If I was anything, I was an agnostic. I needed proof and wasn't getting any. Over many years of study and introspective work, I have come to believe that there probably is a higher power, a God or Spirit that affects human behavior. I have seen too much data in my life that could not be explained any other way, but the scientist in me also sees the possibility that God is simply a creation of the human imagination.

Consider this: In our primitive state, there was so much we could not explain, such as thunder and lightning. We now understand that these are phenomena of the physical world caused by changes in temperature and electrical charges, but to primitive people they were frightening and potentially life-threatening. Primitive people told themselves that this was the work of a higher power that was exerting its strength, and to feel safe, to have some degree of control over the unknown, they created ideas and rules around this higher power: "If God is angry, we must have done something to deserve this." "If I behave in ways to please God, bad things won't happen to me." This gave primitive people some sense of control and understanding of the events. That control made them feel safer. In this model, primitive people created the story of God to soothe their fears; thus, God may have been primitive people's creation, coming from the human Neuroimagination.

In my work as a physician, I see this logic all the time around people's health issues. They believe that if they just behaved differently, if they didn't piss God off, they wouldn't be dealing with their disease. They blame their diseases on negative thoughts or bad karma. The truth is that health crises arise for "good" and "bad" people. You can hedge your bets by living a healthier life, but that in no way means you will be immune to disease.

In many ways, this fear and crisis avoidance may have been the basis for the creation of religion: beliefs and practices to please an unseeable God or gods.

If we apply the concept of neuroplasticity to our ancestors, it would make sense that their brains would remodel to incorporate the God concept into their everyday lives as a way of explaining the unknown, creating the perception of safety in a potentially unsafe world. In essence, through their newly adapted beliefs and behaviors, they remodeled their brains, creating the physical God spot.

It has been demonstrated that a younger brain is more malleable than a brain of an adult, and so if the God concept was introduced at a young age (that thunder—oh, that's just God bowling, my mom told me), the brain's adaptation would be greater and the God concept would be more deeply woven into the structure of the young person's brain, reinforcing religious beliefs and behaviors at a deep, unconscious level. If we expand this discussion to include epigenetics—which theorizes that we alter not only our brain through beliefs and practices but our genes as well—the God concept might be passed down from generation to generation.

As entire societies developed with the God concept incorporated into their daily lives, the brains of those folks would be very different from the brains of their ancestors. Their belief in God and the activity of the God spot change them over time, and their behaviors reflect these changes. These behaviors and beliefs become so well integrated into people's unconscious minds that they can't imagine a world without them.

Our perception of what is real is merely a reflection

of our Neuroimagination. Therefore, God is real in this way, and God affects our lives and behaviors dramatically. As long as we believe that there is a God, we behave as if there is a God, and this shapes our brains and our communities. If this God spot is part of your brain, you are unable to see anything but the existence of God.

Do we have the God spot because it developed as described above, through time and generations, or did God put it there? It's a chicken-or-egg question. We may never know the answer. Did we create the God spot or did God create us?

As to our behaviors and the way we perceive the world, it doesn't matter whether God is inside us or outside us. The effect on our lives and behaviors is the same.

If it is true that we created God with our Neuroimaginations, how can we explain events perceived as miracles? It may be that these events are just things that we can't yet explain through science, as cavemen couldn't explain thunder and lightning, or it may be that there is in fact a God.

I thought about the rattlesnake Cheryl and I had seen on our hike. Was the snake there as a message from God or Spirit, or was it just a sick snake on the side of the path that I interpreted as a message from the divine?

Native American traditions have an interesting take

on these unexplained moments. In many of those traditions, these moments represent the hand of the spirit world reaching into our lives. Spirit is all around us and within us; it is all one. The shaman's role is to bring Spirit in to do the work of healing. The shaman does not heal; the shaman's role is to create a space for Spirit to do the healing. The shaman comes to this role through life experience and practice. A typical shaman's tale details the survival of a major life crisis, often a physical illness that brings the shaman to the brink of death, and a subsequent spiritual awakening. Through this transition, shamans gain access to the healing power of Spirit. In accessing Spirit, there are many experiences and visions that are difficult to explain rationally or scientifically.

In my work, I have seen many things that could not be explained easily or rationally. In one shamanic journey using breathwork, I saw a dreamlike image of the deceased father of a good friend of mine tell my friend that he finally understood what my friend's work had been about and how much he appreciated the work his son had done. After the journey, my friend relayed the same experience. He had seen what I had seen. Somehow we had shared the same vision. Coincidence?

I have seen scenes of abuse that I later confirmed with the individuals involved. I have seen life situations that caused emotional damage that could not be explained but have been confirmed to me by the individuals after the journeys. I have seen the ghostlike spirits of unborn children reaching out to their mothers, who were in the journey process, wanting to be reunited with them, only to find out later that those women had had miscarriages in the past.

All these experiences may be explained through the concept of the Neuroimaginal mind. I may have created them through my own wishes or beliefs or accessed them through some kind of collective unconscious. Although I understand this, it still doesn't feel like an adequate explanation. These events seem more profound.

There have been other remarkable and inexplicable moments in my life when I used shamanic techniques. Kathy, who has always had a healthy skepticism about spiritual events, once asked me to do something remarkable. Her mother was in an intensive care unit in Maryland after a severe health crisis, blood infections, and multiple strokes. She should have been dead but seemed to be hanging on. I was teaching a workshop in Hawaii. Kathy asked me to go visit her mother to find out why she was holding on to life. She obviously was not asking me to fly to Maryland but to journey to her mother by leaving my body, using translocation if you will. I was astonished that my wife asked me to do this, but I knew Kathy wanted her mom to go peacefully and end her suffering, and this moved her to ask for something outside her box.

That night, I used a shamanic journey process to "visit" with Kathy's mother. I closed my eyes and took deep, rapid breaths until I felt myself release from my thoughts of the moment and then slowed my respiration to deep, meditative breathing while focusing my thoughts on Kathy's mom. I began to get an image of her, a bit fuzzy but clear enough to know it was real.

There she was, in a cold intensive care unit bed, with the mechanical sound of the ventilator breathing for her. I saw her body, but the woman I knew as my mother-in-law wasn't in it. The body had no life in it. I looked up, and there she was hovering above her body, a cloud-like, ghostly version of the woman I had known for thirty years. I asked her why she couldn't let go. She looked at me with worry in her eyes and said, "Who will take care of Daddy?" That was what she called my father-in-law. I said, "Mom, we will, don't worry." She giggled and held her hand above her mouth as she often did to hide her teeth and went off with an amazing look of peace and freedom.

I called Kathy the next morning and told her that her

mother had died that night. I knew in my heart that she had let go. Kathy said, "No way; my sisters never called me." Checking, she realized her cell phone had been shut off during the night and that there was a message; her mother had indeed died quietly that night. I cannot explain this with science. I had helped her mother let go and was delighted to tell Kathy that she went with a giggle.

Carl Jung had a series of inexplicable experiences happen to him in 1913. In his dreams, he had images of the streets of his native Switzerland being covered in blood. He then saw floods destroying countless thousands, followed by a barren land where nothing could grow. He thought he was going mad until a few months later when World War I broke out. It was then that he realized that his dreams and visions were premonitions of what was to come.

Over the next few years Jung documented his visions and those of his patients and realized that the phenomenon was not uncommon. Somehow people were tapping into a collective unconscious and accessing information from beyond their bodies. Jung and his patients could visualize and experience things that were not accessible to them through direct human interaction. From this he developed the discipline of transpersonal psychology, a therapeutic approach that includes accessing information from the collective unconscious, much as shamans and religious healers had been doing by accessing God or Spirit for thousands of years.

In the realm of transpersonal psychology, these spiritual events would be explained as shared interhuman events triggered by the connection of our souls. In this language, God may be the combined soul of all beings, the true collective. The explanation then would be that all living beings share an energetic connection and that in certain states all experiences can be shared. It would make sense that in quiet moments such as meditation and in trance moments such as shamanic journeys these interhuman contacts can be experienced more easily. This may be the reason our brains are hardwired to pick up spiritual experiences. It may be why I and many others have accessed information and experiences outside the usual realms of thought. Maybe the God spot is a receiver of information from the collective unconscious.

In my life, there have been many experiences, such as the pennies from heaven and even my experience with the death of Kathy's mom, that I could explain away and tell myself that it was all in my mind. I tend to have a reasonable level of skepticism about these events, as I know the power of the brain to tell itself stories. If I was the only one who experienced an event, I generally interpret it as coming, at least in part, from my Neuroimagination. However, some events leave me without a clue.

Every year for the last fifteen years, my friend Nita and I have taught a weeklong retreat at the Hui Ho'Olana in Hawaii, during which we use the Shamanic Breathwork Process. We do the breathwork in an octagonal wooden building surrounded by a dense tropical forest filled with life: birds sing, geckos "kiss" (a noise that sounds like a small pucker), and leaves rustle. During a particularly rich breathwork session, one of our participants, a physician named Kevin, started to arch his back in pain as if his chest were being pulled upward. He had a disturbing grimace on his face, and I could sense a deep inner trauma. I moved next to him and received an image of a black tarlike substance surrounding and smothering his heart. After many years of doing shamanic work, I have learned that there are times to take actions that may make no logical sense in the usual language of medicine. Many of these techniques come from Native shamanistic teaching and energy healing. In this case, my instincts told me to reach into his chest—energetically—and clear the gunk away. It was gooey-feeling, like moving through a thick liquid, in my hands as I tried to remove it bit by bit. I had some success, but this felt harder than any energy work I had done before. I was getting tired, which is not common. I knew I needed help.

I sat behind him in a meditative pose and asked up to God or Spirit, "Can you help this one?" Within a few seconds, I saw a golden glow and two hands reaching into and around his heart. The arms were covered in white robes, and the hands were gentle and delicate. My inner knowing told me that these were the hands of Jesus (kind of a weird vision for a Jewish guy to have). I could hardly breathe. There was an unending sense of compassion and grace. Tears came to my eyes because this was more beautiful than anything I had ever seen before. Those huge and delicate hands held my friend's heart for about five minutes while I watched in amazement. I did nothing and said nothing but just felt hugely honored to have been a witness to this healing.

After the session one of the other participants asked what had happened to Kevin. This person had seen a golden glow above Kevin's chest. That freaked me out. I equivocated and said that I didn't know what had happened but that it seemed powerful. Then Nita turned to me and said, "What happened with Kevin? There was this massive energy around him."

Now my skepticism was really starting to get shaken.

Although Nita hadn't seen exactly what I had seen, she had seen something significant.

"I was cleaning up this gunk around Kevin's heart and knew that it was too big for me, so I asked for help. I swear that I saw the hands of Jesus come in and heal his heart." I knew my surprise must have shown on my face.

We agreed not to say anything to the other participants, as we wanted them to have their own experience with this, especially Kevin, but we were buzzing with amazement.

On the way back to my cabin, I had a compulsion to call Kathy. I had to share this with her.

"How did you know it was Jesus?" she asked with clear doubt in her voice.

"It was the sandals, the robe, and his name tag that said 'Hi, I'm Jesus. How can I help you?' that gave it away."

She laughed, and I could tell deep down that she was moved and curious. It may have been the tone of my voice, but she knew that something beyond belief had happened.

The next morning at breakfast Kevin asked what I had done to his chest. He said it felt like I had done heart surgery. I brushed it off and mentioned that I had done some energy work on his chest, including pressure, which may have caused some soreness. He then asked me what I had done to his hands. In the middle of both palms were silver-dollar-size bruises that were perfectly round. He also had them on his feet. I had heard of stigmata before but had never seen them or, frankly, believed in them.

"What did you feel during the breathwork?" I asked, eager to know what he had experienced.

"I felt like my heart was being held—no, healed—by a something gentle and beautiful."

This made the experience far more real for me. If Kevin had seen Jesus, it would have been possible that he somehow could have created the stigmata unconsciously. The fact that he hadn't connected the experience with Jesus, yet spontaneously developed marks on his hands and feet that he did not interpret as stigmata, was profound. He was, in research terms, blinded to the effect, and the outcome was documented and witnessed by other observers.

Up to that point I had tried to remain skeptical. Maybe I wanted to hand Kevin over to Jesus for healing. Maybe in that trancelike state of breathwork that effect is what I created; however, I knew I hadn't touched Kevin's hands. That blew me away. I had no way of explaining this through neurophysiology or science, yet here was my colleague with stigmata on both hands and feet!

I sat and breathed in the wonder of the event, stunned, amazed, and hugely honored to have been there. This was a miracle—I had witnessed the healing work of Jesus.

I knew enough just to sit there and watch as Kevin showed his stigmata to the group. I did not take credit or insert myself into the story; it was not about me. This was one bite of a sandwich that I would enjoy forever.

As my connection with God or Spirit increased through these events, I began to realize that there was no need to try to control life. All I could do was enjoy the ride as life occurred in all its suffering and joy. After all, if there *is* a God or Spirit outside of us, how much control do we actually have? I realized that my little plans meant nothing in the grand scheme of things. I had no control when it came to the big picture of life.

So why do we need to feel that we are in control? It's simple. For most people, control equals a perception of safety. Think back to our cave-dwelling ancestors and thunder: If we understand it, we can control it; if we can control it, it won't hurt us. We use the same kind of magical thinking about our health: If I can control all of my risk factors for disease, I won't get sick. Unfortunately, this is a fallacy. We all know people who lived healthy lives and died young, and we all know people who smoked heavily and ate poorly and lived to a ripe old age.

Let me tell you a story that is based on an old Chinese tale. A sixty-year-old man who has never owned a car wins a new car in a fund-raising lottery. All his friends tell him how lucky he is because now he can visit his kids more often and go to the market or movies whenever he wants. His only response is, "Lucky? Maybe yes, maybe no." A few weeks later, he has an accident in the new car and ends up in the hospital. His friends tell him that this is a tragedy, that he should never have driven and how unlucky it was that he won the new car. His response is, "Unlucky? Maybe yes, maybe no." While he is in the hospital, there is an electrical fire in his house. If he had been there, he surely would have died. His friends tell him how lucky he is to have been in the hospital and that he will recover from the accident but that he would be dead if he had been at home. His response is, "Lucky? Maybe yes, maybe no."

This story can go on forever, but the important message is that we really don't know what the long-term outcome of any event or choice will be. We base choices on our Neuroimaginal projections of outcomes. In doing so we may hedge our bets on the basis of past experience, but we really don't know what will happen. How many great ideas and how many business plans fail?

How much control do we actually have in the big picture of our lives? I would say very little, if any. This can be either disturbing or liberating. It is disturbing and scary if lack of control makes you feel unsafe or if fear prevents you from taking risks and trying new things. It squashes creativity and prevents you from living fully.

However, having no control can be liberating if you can relax and accept this concept. Living life this way leads to wonder and curiosity; it is the basis of creativity and personal growth. This also decreases fear of death, as death is not within our control. It is the ultimate unknown. Just live life, do your best, and enjoy the moments that life brings.

I am not suggesting that you throw all caution to the wind and just walk around saying, "I have no control." Societal and moral rules were created to enhance our capacities to live together and minimize harm to others. After all, I am not ruling out the idea of heaven or hell, so hedge your bets in the direction that feels right to you.

I do know that the more in touch we are with the oneself and the more detached we become from the day-to-day self of worrying, the more open we can be to change and creativity. The more you can accept this, the less fear you will have.

If you can accept this lack of control, you can accept anything that arises and accept that it may be good or bad and you won't know for some time to come, if ever. Therefore, nothing begins to appear as bad. Life, as Helen Keller said, can be a "daring adventure," and all events can become learning experiences.

You get to choose the world you want to live in. It can be a house of fear and constriction or a house of mystery and creativity. Do you choose anger or compassion about your frailties and the frailties of others? In your world will it be the fear of death or the joy of life? It is that simple.

SIXTEEN

Zuzu's Petals

Some days there won't be a song in your heart. Sing anyway.
—*Emory Austin*

In the classic film *It's a Wonderful Life,* George Bailey, played by Jimmy Stewart, is feeling that his life has meant nothing. On a cold winter's night, after a terrible financial mishap, he gets drunk, gets into a barroom fight, and yells at his wife. He gets mad at his daughter Zuzu, who had wanted him to fix her flower, which was losing its petals. George stuffs the petals in his pockets and leaves the house. At the end of this long, hopeless night he ends up on a bridge, ready to jump into the icy waters below, feeling worthless and angry at himself for yelling at everyone he loves. He no longer wants to live.

An angel, Clarence, comes to him and shows how miserable his family and his town would have become if not for the small loving things he had done throughout his life. His wife would have been a frightened spinster, his town an economic mess, his brother dead, his friends miserable, his children unborn.

Bailey comes to realize how much he has meant to others and how rich his life has really been. This is confirmed when he reaches into his pocket and finds the petals of Zuzu's flower. In that moment, he knows he has a second chance at life.

Like George Bailey, we all have the opportunity to remake our lives if we just remember what meaning and purpose we already have. We can simply reach into our pocket and find the pieces of our life that remind us that this is in fact a wonderful life.

> *No man is poor who has friends.*
> —*Clarence the Angel in* It's a Wonderful Life

For me Zuzu's petals have been the relationships I have developed, the children I have raised, and the work I have done. The petals have been the support of my family and friends. They are also the e-mails, cards, and letters from friends around the world after my diagnosis about how much they appreciate me and my work; notes about how I changed lives, saved marriages, and inspired careers. My life has had meaning. I am grateful that I have had the chance to be this person, on this planet, at this time. I am grateful that I could receive this love and support. I know that if I die today, this has been a wonderful life. Relationships are always the main ingredients of most people's sandwiches, and you could say that gratitude is the bread that holds it all together.

Most of us experience gratitude in our lives around gifts, friends, kind acts, or sometimes just a good meal, but how much time do we spend each day consciously being grateful for these things or these moments? Rarely do we make gratitude a practice.

The daily practice of gratitude shifts your focus onto the parts of life that you appreciate. You still see and manage the difficult areas of your life, but your emotional focus shifts to gratefulness. When we practice gratitude each day, life becomes sweet regardless of our life circumstances.

During my cancer treatment a friend of mine, Mark, in North Carolina and I had a late-night text message conversation that led to us toasting each other three thousand miles apart. It was one of my last tastes of great scotch shared with a dear friend. It was a delight to be with him through technology in my moments of fatigue.

Nothing fancy, nothing dramatic, just simple friendship. Simple moment, simple gratitude.

An event that changed my view of so-called bucket lists occurred in the middle of my treatment. Another friend named Mark; his wife, Anna; and their family came to visit us from Pittsburgh on one of my chemo breaks. Knowing that my life might be shorter than expected and knowing my love of rock 'n' roll, he asked me one day what band I would most like to see before I died. Laughingly, I said the Beatles (I knew I might have to wait until after I died for that one!).

When I was a seven-year-old sitting on the floor, two feet from a round black-and-white TV, watching the Beatles on the *Ed Sullivan Show,* my life changed. The energy, vibrancy, and passion coming out of the tiny TV speaker resonated through my little body, creating a passion for rock 'n' roll that still lives.

Mark said, "Would you like to meet Paul McCartney?" I said, "Sure," knowing that this was an impossible task for a guy who is not in the music industry and a difficult one even for those who are connected. He called me a month later to tell me that he was working on it and had a plan. He had gotten in touch with Paul's pilot, whom he knew from Pittsburgh, and was trying to make it happen.

I was laughing my head off with delight. Although meeting Sir Paul would have been on my bucket list, I had something better: a friend who would go well out of his way to do something to make me happy. Just knowing this was a huge petal in my pocket.

I no longer have a bucket list. I have love in my life. This is far greater than seeing the Pyramids, climbing mountains, eating Thai food in Thailand, or any other physical activity that might be fun to experience. I am loved and I have loved. My bucket list is complete.

I believe we are all born with the capacity for gratitude, but many times we get in our own way. A common example of this is pessimism and perfectionism. Pessimists and perfectionists may have things to be grateful for in life but will rapidly find a reason why it is not right or perfect or how it could have been better. Their Neuro-imaginal minds search for mistakes or flaws. In doing so, they immediately jump to the negative without enjoying even a brief moment of gratitude. "Yes, but . . ." is their language. They can't enjoy a sandwich because it has too much mayonnaise or too little lettuce or the bread is too hard or too soft.

On the other end of the spectrum are those who ignore difficulty until their lives fall apart. I often see this in people with significant spiritual lives and practices. They blind themselves to life's realities by diving deeper into their practices: "If I just meditate and do my yoga, this will all go away." I have seen many people who are not aware of themselves or the harm they do to others and use spiritual practice to avoid their real lives.

My friend Nita and I refer to this as spiritual bypass. People use spiritual practices and beliefs to excuse the harmful things they do to others and avoid or "bypass" who they truly are. Gurus and priests do this unconsciously to avoid the dark aspects of their personalities. This is how child abuse and sexual affairs can occur among religious leaders. They haven't dared to look at their shadows. They can enjoy their sandwiches, but while they eat, the ceiling falls down on them. Ignorance is not always bliss.

Gratitude practice means facing reality, gaining awareness of the many aspects of yourself: your inner self, your one-self, your subpersonalities and those of the people around you. It means understanding and embracing your shadow. It means letting go of a need to control yourself and others, it means growing compassion for those who have hurt you, it means being aware of the difficult parts of your life and still being able to reach into your pocket on a dark, snowy night, just before you leap from a bridge, to find a small, innocent petal. Gratitude is the ultimate expression of hope.

A healthy practice of gratitude is simple. You don't need to whitewash the bad, just remind yourself of the good now and then. Remember, what you look for is what you find.

A simple way to do this that has worked well for me is to keep a pad or journal at your bedside and each night write down three things you are grateful for that happened that day. It can be simple things such as a great meal, a good joke, or just being happy that you ran into someone you liked. As you develop this practice, you will find that you begin to look for things to write each day and that instead of looking for things that are wrong in the world, you start focusing on things that are right. After doing this for about three weeks, you will start to notice a difference. You are remodeling your brain to be grateful, even optimistic.

Another simple practice has helped me immensely. It was developed by an organization called HeartMath and is called Quick Coherence®. The core of this process is to breathe very deeply and slowly and think of a positive emotion. You SHIFT your breathing, as if the long slow breaths were coming in and around your heart, while you ACTIVATE the positive emotion. Something that you are grateful for works well. Hold this state of positive emotion and do deep, slow breathing for at least one minute when you first learn the practice. The SHIFT in breathing balances your nervous system and puts it in a more relaxed state. The ACTIVATION of a positive emotion retrains your brain to think optimistically and harmoniously.

This combination of breathing and positive emotion is extraordinarily effective at reducing stress and building gratitude. You can expand this practice by thinking of people you love and things you love to do. Almost any positive emotion works well.

This practice has made a profound difference in even the most mundane aspects of my life. It has helped me control anger and find gratitude even in difficult moments. I was teaching in the Washington, DC, area for Kaiser and was to fly to Wisconsin that night to teach at 9 A.M. the next day. In the middle of my class, I received a text message from United Airlines that my flight had been canceled. I shifted my breathing and focused on the people in my workshop whom I was fond of (positive emotion). SHIFT and ACTIVATE. This calmed me right down and allowed me to keep teaching. I wasn't deluding myself; I was enjoying the group.

After the program ended, I called United and asked if there was an alternative way to get to the Milwaukee area by the next morning. They told me that the only flight I could use was out of Baltimore Washington International Airport and was going to Chicago and that I would have to drive the rest of the way. Although this meant driving in rush hour traffic and getting into Wisconsin quite late, I shifted my breathing and activated gratitude that I would at least get there. It was still a pain in the backside, but I shifted my focus to the final outcome, toward the positive, which avoided adding anxiety and frustration to a challenging situation. SHIFT and ACTIVATE.

When I got to the airport check-in desk, there was no one there. It was now about forty minutes before the last flight (mine), so the ticketing personnel had left. I rang the bell a few times and shifted my breathing. The positive emotion I came up with was to think of my friends Harry and Cheryl, who live nearby. My worst-case scenario was that I was stuck there and would call Harry and Cheryl and see if they wanted to spend the evening together. I could then get on an early flight the next day. SHIFT and ACTIVATE.

I finally got the attention of one of the United personnel, and she told me that she didn't have me on their list. SHIFT and ACTIVATE—dinner with Harry and

Cheryl. Her supervisor noted that I was a gold flier and that they would get me to Chicago, but the only seat was a middle seat in the last row, not comfortable at all. SHIFT and ACTIVATE. I would still get there.

Fortunately, I ended up sitting next to a guy in his thirties who wanted to open a blues club in Maryland. We had a great two hours together talking about music and swapping iPods. It turned out to be fun. SHIFT and ACTIVATE.

Although I now had a two-hour drive to Wisconsin from Chicago, I called my wife, who was at our son's baseball playoff game. She began to give me a play-by-play of the game and proceeded to pass the phone to all our friends in the stands, who continued giving me the play-by-play action. Sports radio from a game over two thousand miles away, with my wife as the lead announcer, is a moment that I will never forget.

What could have been a miserable travel experience turned out to be fun. Twenty years ago I would have been pissed off at United Airlines and grumbled through the whole experience. Now I just SHIFT and ACTIVATE—deal with what is before me and move on.

In coping with my cancer, this simple technique has been very effective. While sitting for six hours, getting chemo and feeling like shit, I can shift my focus to how the chemo is killing the cancer cells and change my attitude about the treatment. I used this while lying on the radiation table, SHIFTing my breathing and ACTIVATing the image of my cancer cells shrinking away. Pain becomes hope.

Through this technique I have learned to enjoy being home even while feeling sick. Instead of whining that I am not working and earning an income, I SHIFT, ACTIVATE, and enjoy good movies. Instead of whining that I can't stand up for rock shows at the Fillmore, I SHIFT and ACTIVATE and enjoy earlier, seated shows. Life goes on; it's just different now, and a good sandwich is still a good sandwich.

Gratitude has been built and strengthened with these simple daily practices. I can still focus on and manage problems in my life. I just give myself a break every so often with gratitude. Just SHIFT and ACTIVATE.

My father taught me to do work that I love. He always said that I would spend more time at work than anyplace else. I use the gratitude practice to focus on the parts of my work that excite me and give me the most pleasure. This has helped me develop my career in ways that give me joy and passion for my work. I have grown my career with gratitude for what I get to do each day. When I had to stop working, I shifted to gratitude that I could be home with Kathy each day. I found local volunteer work and blogging to feed the work-oriented part of my soul. Gratitude helps keep life fluid. Life is about flexibility; death is about rigidity. It's called rigor mortis for a reason.

I also practice gratitude in a much more profound way. On a very cold winter's morning about fifteen years ago, lying in bed at five-thirty in the morning, instead of getting up to meditate in the living room, which I have done for years, I decided to meditate in bed. That morning I chose to do a meditation on love, so I stretched out my arm and Kathy rolled over onto my chest. I meditated for forty-five minutes on how much love there is in my life and how grateful I am for it. Kathy seemed to purr in her sleep. For fifteen years, this has been my morning routine, thirty to forty-five minutes of love before getting up. I know that I am retraining my brain toward unconditional love. I also know that I am generating deep gratitude for my life, which is very rich and meaningful, and I also believe that by sending love to her in this way, I can affect Kathy's life positively. What a great way to start a day: gratitude and love—my bread and sandwich ingredients in one tasty bite.

SEVENTEEN

Love Soup

Ever has it been that love knows not its own
depth until the hour of separation.
—Khalil Gibran

Kathy's response to my cancer has been varied. At times she was the doctor: "Do this; don't do that." At times she was the caregiver, getting me anything she thought I needed. Occasionally she would just hold me. That was the hardest part for her.

Holding her weak and sickly husband—helping me to the bathroom to vomit, watching me struggle in pain to get out of bed—was at times almost unbearable for her. I looked like a cancer guy: sallow skin, knit cap, sweatshirt and pants, thin and weak. Sometimes I know I looked like death itself.

It was impossible for her to work a full day at the

clinic, come home to attend to me, and then face the fact that I might be dying. She did the first two very well. She was working, cooking, cleaning, shopping, and caring for me in all the ways she could manage, but she struggled just to hold me. Kathy's way of showing love is by doing; my way of showing love is by being. Neither of our needs could be fully met.

Kathy became the queen of soup. She and Cheryl love soup and can eat it 24/7. I don't love soup. There are a few soups that I enjoy, especially hot and sour soup and French onion soup, but a stomach bathed in chemo and getting radiation daily would not do well with either of them. In the course of a two-week period, Kathy made seven different soups as I gently reminded her that I didn't like soup before I was sick and being sick did not enhance my taste for it. The queen of soup persisted. Her doing for me was her way of loving me even if it didn't meet my needs.

One night, during the period when I was getting chemo and radiation, I was profoundly weak, sick, and exhausted. I needed to be held. I stumbled out of bed, nauseous, and worked my way into the living room, where Kathy was watching *Private Practice*. Kathy loves medical shows. This has always struck me as funny, as they are usually ridiculously artificial: The doctors are all good-looking, the diagnoses are always correct, and pediatricians do heart surgery. Even Kathy admits that they are silly, but they are good escapist fare. She spends her days seeing patients and then comes home to watch other doctors take care of patients.

On this night I needed to be held. I didn't need food, I didn't need water, and I especially didn't need soup. I was exhausted but couldn't bear going to sleep alone.

In a weakened voice I asked, "Come to bed and hold me until I fall asleep."

"I want to watch *Private Practice*," she said.

"Come hold me, please, just until I fall asleep. You can watch *Private Practice* in the bedroom."

"No," she insisted, "I want to watch it here."

I got angry: "TiVo it. TiVo every fucking episode, and when I die, you can watch them all." She was shocked and turned away from me, crying.

I went to bed angry. I didn't need soup. I didn't need television. I needed my wife to hold me. Throughout the next day I was still pissed off. Why couldn't she just hold me when I needed her to? As I sat with this and moved past the anger, I began to realize that holding me meant being with me while I was sick. Holding me meant suffering with me. Holding me meant that her husband was dying.

The next night, soup in hand, I asked her if this was true. She agreed. After a full day of working, cooking, and cleaning, having to be reminded of my mortality was just too much to handle. She needed to escape it all through TV.

I soon learned that Kathy had her own way of dealing with my dying. She would go out for a run, and with each footfall, a tear would shake loose from her eyes. She ran until she could cry no more, pounding her pain into the pavement with each exhausting step until she could return home to become a caregiver all over again. We both had to deal with my dying in our own way, and even though those ways were often at odds, we learned to accept our differences, although at times it still saddened me.

This last New Year's Eve we went to a small party with old friends and came home and had a little champagne together while sitting on the couch. Kathy started to cry.

"Last New Year's Eve I sat on the couch, watching the ball in Times Square drop. You had already fallen asleep, and I sat here crying, knowing that I would be spending every New Year's Eve for the rest of my life alone, without you."

She had never shared that with me. I was very happy to postpone her vision, at least for one year.

Over time and as I have recovered, she has become much more able just to be with me, to hold me when I need it. I want hugs, not drugs (or soup), I tell her.

My cancer has been much harder for Kathy than it has been for me. I can make choices about what I eat and what supplements I take and about keeping myself active, which gives me some degree of control over the situation. My wife has no power at all. She can't control my behaviors or my choices of treatment, and she certainly can't control the cancer. For a strong woman who prefers to be in control, this at times is more than she can bear.

I soon accepted that the only thing I could do to make it better was to live, and I was already trying to do that. I could keep participating in life, be in touch with my inner husband, and love her for who she is, not who I wish she was. I have even learned to sit with her on the couch and hold her while she watches medical shows.

The process of dealing with dying has led to some conversations that never would have happened before. We have laughingly designed my funeral, where I write the eulogies for our friends and family members to deliver. The plan is for my friend Ronna to play "Hit the Road Jack" on guitar as everyone lines up to do tequila shots, and then a funk band plays while everyone drunkenly dances. If you gotta go, do it in style.

On two of my chemo breaks (you get a month between rounds of chemo so that the treatment doesn't kill
you before the cancer does), we went down to San José
del Cabo, Mexico, just to lie on the beach, read, and walk
into town each evening for dinner and ice pops. It was
a way to just have time together. The food was great,
and since I had come off chemo, my appetite was back.
More than that, I hadn't had alcohol in months and
really missed a good tequila buzz. My first margarita in
months was heaven. My liver also hadn't seen alcohol in
months, and I was a cheap date, completely ripped on
one drink and savoring every moment of it.

As we were lying on a round bedlike mattress together in an open-air hut on a two-mile stretch of beach,
I asked Kathy, "If I die, will you date other men?"

I really wanted to let her know that it would be okay
and that I wouldn't mind at all. I want her to be happy
and have fun for the rest of her life, even if it's without me.

She turned, looked at me very seriously, and said,
"No, you've ruined me for other men."

I thought she was teasing me. "Come on, I'm not joking. Would you?"

She looked at me with what I knew was deep love in
her eyes. "I'm not joking. We have such a great marriage,
and trying to create this all over again would be more

than I want to do. You know how shy I am. I've had one great marriage, and that's enough for me."

I melted. This was the sweetest thing I had ever heard from her, and I knew her well enough to know that it was true. I felt the same way, too. The truth is that our marriage has been great even if it has not always been easy. There have been challenges, struggles, missteps, and misalignments, and not just about soup. Still, this relationship was worth a lifetime of love no matter how long or short.

Deep down, I know that if I die, men will pursue her. She is sweet, sexy, and a joy to be with. She's a baseball fan, is very fit, looks hot in biking shorts, and loves life. Any man would be lucky to have her, and many men will try, I'm sure. I hope they do, for her sake. She deserves the pleasure of life and being pursued. I only hope they are as loving to her as I have tried to be.

We had another conversation recently that surprised me. I realized that when I die, I don't want to be stuck underground somewhere without her. I asked Kathy if it would be okay if I was cremated and kept in a box at home, and when she dies, we could ask the kids to cremate her and we could be buried together. She cried and said that it was the most romantic thing she had ever heard. These are not the usual conversations couples in their fifties have. I am grateful that we've had the opportunity to have them.

I encourage you to have these conversations with your loved ones, difficult or otherwise. Don't wait until it is too late. It is a blessing to be with each other this way.

Over time and through cancer we have opened up to each other in ways that I couldn't have imagined. Facing death has moved us even closer to loving each other unconditionally.

Unconditional love is not easy in partner relationships. Being together is often filled with subtle conditions. "I love you when you do X" is a condition. "I hate you when Y" is a condition. In unconditional love, we may hate or love it when our partner does something, but our love for him or her is constant. Most parents experience this with their children. I even hear parents say, "I don't always like them, but I always love them." That is unconditional love.

In our relationship, there are certainly moments when Kathy does things that aggravate me, and rest assured, I know I do things that aggravate her. One simple tool I have learned to use when she angers me is to ask myself, "Do I love her anyhow?" For over thirty years, the answer has been yes. This has helped me more than anything to move toward unconditionally loving her. Cancer has made small arguments in our lives even smaller. It really doesn't matter if the dishes aren't clean. What matters is that we are here for each other.

True love, which grows over time, may not just be a psychological, cognitive experience; there is something deeper and shared going on. There is a growing scientific literature on the physiological and energetic interactions between people.

Rollin McCraty, HeartMath's director of research, has done work in this area. He first measured the electromagnetic field around individuals in different mood states and demonstrated that there are clear, reproducible patterns of electromagnetic energy that appear with different moods. If a person is angry or hostile, there is one clear pattern; if the same person is in a loving state, a very different pattern of electromagnetic energy is created. Is it possible that we can detect these changes radiating from another person and respond to this energy? There is every reason to believe this is possible. Reptiles have been shown to respond to changes in electromagnetic fields. They walk toward loving energy and away from angry energy. It wouldn't be a huge stretch to believe that we would do the same thing.

Rollin has also demonstrated that when two people

are touching, the EKG (measures heart rhythm) of one person is detected in the EEG (measures brain waves) of the other person, showing that one person's heart rhythm has the potential to affect another person's brain wave patterning. He is, as of this writing, working on a project to demonstrate the same effect between a baby's heart rhythm and the mother's brain waves when they are touching.

Linda Russek and Gary Schwartz at the University of Arizona have demonstrated this effect in adults who are not touching. In their experiment, they had two subjects sit in close proximity to each other in an electrically isolated environment. They can actually cause alteration in each other's heart rhythms and brain waves just by being close to each other.

In this study, the first effect was a synchronization of the two people's heart rhythms. The hearts began to beat as one, literally. Shortly afterward, those individuals begin to effect change in each other's brain waves. Their brain function begins to find a middle ground of activity; in essence, the two people become of one mind. I'm sure you have seen this effect in couples over time. The longer they are together, sleeping in proximity, the more they begin to think and act like each other. Therefore, when I am holding Kathy and loving her each morning, I am affecting her brain function and physiology. We are becoming one energetically, physiologically, and emotionally.

It may be that love is an interpersonal energetic experience. We might even consider that a couple cocreates a Neuroimaginal world together as a loving single entity. With the concept of epigenetics, it may be that their love alters the individual's genetic makeup, and thus this love can be passed on to their children psychologically, energetically, and genetically and to their children after them. You become immortal through the love you generate. The Beatles may have had it right: In the end the love we take may in fact be equal to the love we make.

Love may be a many-splendored and complex neurophysiologic, interhuman construct, but most important, love of family and friends brings magic and joy to our lives. Love brings gratitude and a sense of life's fullness. Love is the filling of life's sandwich.

Our love can continue for many generations even when we can't, but even so there are moments that we will miss. I had come to peace with most things, except one.

Cheryl and her boyfriend, Lee, have been together for four years. She loves him, he loves her, and Kathy and I have embraced him in our family. Through this journey, he has been there for Cheryl and also for Will. We had for the last two years assumed that they would get married, but maybe not soon enough for me to be there.

Cheryl is and always will be my little girl, and I want to be there to see that moment of joy. I want to hold Kathy's hand while our little girl takes her vows of love and commitment. I can imagine it. I can see the tear running down my cheek. I want to walk her down the aisle and hold her in my arms while we dance, just as I held her for the first time when she was born. It's one of those not-to-be-missed moments in a person's life.

Cheryl and I were sitting on a wooden bench at Stinson Beach watching the sun set. I put my arm around her and squeezed her a little as the sun drifted behind the clouds.

"Mom tells me that you two were talking about where to buy a diamond ring." I tried to quell my excitement.

"Lee doesn't trust himself to buy the right one," Cheryl responded. "So Mom and I are going to look."

"I never told you this, but the only thing I knew that I would regret missing if I died soon was your wedding. I didn't want to affect your choice about whether to get married or when."

I had finally said the last thing that for me was left unsaid. Whether I made it to the wedding or not, I was satisfied.

I drew her closer, and we watched the sun disappear into the ocean.

> *Love doesn't make the world go 'round. Love is what makes the ride worthwhile.*
> —*Franklin P. Jones*

EIGHTEEN

Living and Dying Outside the Box

We create the world we live in. Some of us have large, comfortable homes with room to grow, and others have tiny, boxlike apartments that keep us feeling small and confined. When I was younger, I lived in a Neuro-imaginal box of depression and anxiety where smart people became doctors or lawyers and relationships were like those idealized stories presented to me daily on television and in movies: Good people get good things, love is pure and romantic, and bad guys always get it in the end. At that time, I believed that was all there was to life. I had no way of seeing outside that limited worldview. It was my truth.

When I lived in such a small box, I couldn't imagine any other world or life. I reinforced my limited world over and over by surrounding myself with people who shared my views, passions, and opinions. I defined myself by the world I had created.

I had no desire to leave the little box I lived in, because there was enough comfort, security, and success for me to believe that everything was fine. I came up with justifications for why I couldn't change. I had responsibilities to my wife and kids, to my work. I had invested so many years to build this life and career that the fear of change was greater than my desire to change. Maintaining the status quo was just enough to get by, and I told myself good stories of a successful life to avoid thinking about change. I had solid defense mechanisms.

I was a physician with a wife, children, and a thriving practice. Everything was supposed to be great, but a restlessness began to grow inside me. This restlessness became anxiety and dissatisfaction, and although I wouldn't have used this terminology then, my soul began to call out to me for what it needed: a new self, a new world, something larger. My desire to change began to exceed my fear of change.

I started to explore other options and ask other people about their experiences. People around me who had changed their worlds told me, "Oh, it's easy; I did it. And look how happy I am now. All you need to do is. . . ." I thought that they just didn't understand how hard change would be for me. I was a successful doctor. They hadn't lived my life; they weren't me.

In retrospect, these people had made substantial changes in their lives, but in doing so they forgot what it was like to be stuck in a world of limitations. For them, changing their world seemed so easy, a no-brainer, and of such great value that they wouldn't have it any other way.

As a physician, I have seen so many women wanting a second child after swearing up and down during their first delivery that they would never do it again. Then something magical happens—the presence of a beautiful child, a rush of oxytocin (the bonding hormone), the first birthday, the undeniable cuteness of a baby learning to walk and talk as if by magic, and the memory of the painful birth process fades away. They forget the swelling, the pain, the sleepless nights, and the sutures. They forget the struggle.

Birthing a new life, scratching your way out of a confining box, is very much the same; the freedom and expansiveness at the other end make you forget how traumatic and difficult the work of escaping was. Today I can't imagine living my old life, but I can say that leaving it behind was not easy. I have not forgotten totally the pain of delivery.

But pain always seems to push us until vision starts

to pull us. In my thirties, the pain of living in my depressed and anxious little box finally surpassed my desire for safety, and I began to scratch away at the lining of the box in which I was stuck. For years, I didn't even know where I was going. I just knew that my old world wasn't enough. I scratched away at that box with simple tools: meditation, exercise, rock 'n' roll, love, and therapy. I had no idea what I would find outside the walls of that box. I only knew that it was too painful to live inside it anymore. I was living the life I was supposed to live, but my soul was withering.

So I scratched away each morning, each evening, and each and every day until a small streak of light started to shine through. The wall had become just thin enough for me to know that there was something outside this prison of my own making. After I could see that small glimmer of hope, the effort started to feel worthwhile and change became possible. Inspired, I scratched some more.

After years of scratching, struggle, introspection, and disruption in relationships, the thin opening in my small box became wide enough for me to step out. What I found was a scary, unknown place where all my old emotions and thoughts lived but where they were now accompanied by a new worldview in which thoughts and emotions were just of the moment, not the definition of myself.

This new world I had entered, this new home, was a place of transcendence, anger, depression, and joy, and I had to deal with it all. There was no shield except love. Somehow, without being aware of it, I had created a new home for myself. It was a safe place both to grow in and from which to venture out into the risky unknown. From this new home, life became an adventure in which difficulty was just something to dive into. Every time I did dive in, I came out stronger than before. I came out refreshed and renewed.

This new house of my own creation has changed and now has many rooms. I have built it over many years with my practices of meditation, prayer, therapy, and journeywork, and it continues to expand.

This home has a room called depression where I can sit after struggling to walk up our small hill because my postradiation lungs are burned, coarse remnants of the pink, healthy tissue they once were. In this room I sit and listen to Jackson Browne's "Late for the Sky" and acknowledge what I've lost.

This house has a room called anger where the frenetic energy of punk rock pushes me to flail about until I collapse, usually of exhaustion, expunging anger at those who have hurt me.

This house has a room called joy where Patti Smith's "People Have the Power" is cranked up to eleven on the volume dial, where I laugh, jump, and let tears of pure happiness flow.

This house has a room called love where "God Only Knows" by the Beach Boys plays 24/7 and where I sit and feel the petals of gratitude in my pocket.

This house has a room where my family dances together to Johnny Clegg's "Cruel, Crazy, Beautiful World" and I hold my daughter while hearing Joseph Arthur's "In the Sun."

This house has a room called peace where I meditate and Tibetan bowls ring in their sweet, harmonious tones and overtones, incense burns, and the world of today disappears in the silence of all that is bigger than me.

This house has a room called busy-ness, where a playlist of Springsteen, the Stones, the Beatles, John Prine, the Replacements, NRBQ, and many others are my welcome sound track to a life of doing.

This house has a kitchen where my friends and family gather and create warmth. My dad sings Sinatra as we make sandwiches together—many breads, many fillings, much love.

This house has a room called death where some day—maybe this year, maybe in five years, maybe when I am seventy-eight—I will go to lie down and this body will stop and some version of "I" will rest at last. But the music will play on.

I built this house with practice, experience, and love. It took years of work. It didn't exist before me, and it may not be there once I cease to be.

You too can build a house of your choosing. Like any labor of love, it takes time, patience, and practice. Even if you only have time left to redecorate one room in your existing house, it's worth the effort.

If you are confined inside four small walls, it is impossible to see what lies outside. When you are inside a box of pain, scratch away at the walls. When you are inside a box of depression, scratch away. A box of perfectionism, scratch away. A box of self-pity, scratch away at those walls as if your life depended on it. Because it does. You won't know where you are going, or how to get there, or what it will look like on the other side. But if there is pain or worry or unhappiness, scratch away at the walls that imprison you—scratch away with prayer, meditation, yoga, exercise, laughter, art, movement, gratitude, acceptance, and love. Scratch away with the knowledge that there is so much more to life than what we imagine it to be. There is so much more to death than what we imagine it to be. And there is so much more to living and loving and being than can be seen from inside our little walled-in world. If you choose not to, there is no one else to blame.

I know many patients and many friends who have used these simple gifts to move away from abusive parents, addicted families, and poverty and into a new life. And I have known many who have used these simple gifts to face death squarely and move beyond fear. Some call them amazing. I call them persistent. The pain of staying where they were at some point exceeded the fear of leaving. Their souls demanded to be heard, and they answered the call. Just as I did.

We all have this capacity, we can all learn the necessary tools, and we all have God or Spirit and the shaman within us. We just need to begin to practice, to scratch away at the old Neuroimaginal world we have created and build ourselves a new home.

Patti Smith was right. People do have the power.

Facing my mortality, chemotherapy, radiation, and especially the inability to help those whom I love has made this the most challenging period of my life so far, but simultaneously, I have felt more gratitude and more freedom and peace and life than ever before.

Someday you will face your own mortality. At that moment, I hope you see that your life has been well led, that you hold no regrets, and that you have loved well. On that day, I hope that for you, it has become a good day to die.

ABOUT THE AUTHOR

Lee Lipsenthal, M.D., was an internationally recognized leader, teacher, and author in the fields of integrative medicine and physician wellness. He was the medical director with Dean Ornish of the Preventive Medicine Research Institute in Sausalito, California, for ten years, and has also served as president of the American Board of Integrative Holistic Medicine and on the American Medical Association's Physician Wellness Committee. Through his years in the medical profession, Dr. Lipsenthal observed that the health, morale, and work satisfaction of many physicians were often worse than that of their patients. Inspired by his personal and professional experience, he developed the "Finding Balance in a Medical Life" program, which has been adapted by major medical groups and is being delivered at medical schools and residency programs nationwide.

Lee Lipsenthal died in September 2011. His wife, Kathy, who is also a physician, and his two children live in California.

Dr. Lee Lipsenthal

AUGUST 13, 1957–SEPTEMBER 20, 2011

The world's light has dimmed a little
in losing you, Lee.

You were a true gift to us all.